The

TDOS
Syndrome

The
TDOS
Syndrome

When Toxicity, Nutritional Deficiency, Overweight, and Stress (TDOS) Collide to Threaten Our Health

Peter Greenlaw

WITH NICHOLAS MESSINA, MD, AND DREW GREENLAW

SelectBooks, Inc.
New York

The TDOS Syndrome® is a trademark of Peter Greenlaw.

This edition published by SelectBooks, Inc.
For information address SelectBooks, Inc., New York, New York.

First Edition

ISBN 978-1-59079-410-4

Library of Congress Cataloging-in-Publication Data

Names: Greenlaw, Peter, author.│Messina, Nicholas, author.│Greenlaw, Drew, author.
Title: The TDOS syndrome : how toxicity, nutritional deficiency, overweight, and stress collide to threaten our health / Peter Greenlaw with Nicholas Messina, MD, and Drew Greenlaw.
Description: First edition.│New York : SelectBooks, [2017]│Series: The Greenlaw report series
Identifiers: LCCN 2016030730│ISBN 9781590794104 (paperback)
Subjects: LCSH: Environmental toxicology.│Environmental health.
Classification: LCC RA1226 .G74 2017│DDC 615.9/02--dc23 LC record available at https://lccn.loc.gov/2016030730

Manufactured in the United States of America
10 9 8 7 6 5 4 3 2 1

I want to dedicate this book to all the people who are so desperately searching for ways to improve their quality of life.

If we can help one person in fulfilling the potential to have a high quality of life, then we have been justly rewarded.

This book is here to make you aware of a health problem. In science, if you cannot identify the totality of a problem, you cannot come up with effective solutions.

To the potential of achieving this in all of us.

THE GREENLAW REPORT SERIES

The TDOS Syndrome
When Toxicity, Nutritional Deficiency, Overweight, and Stress
(TDOS) Collide to Threaten Our Health

TDOS Solutions
Fighting Toxicity, Nutritional Deficiency,
Overweight, and Stress (TDOS) Syndrome

Contents

A Note to the Reader

Please note that what I have named the "TDOS Syndrome" is not a disease. This book contains academic and scientific considerations and not medical prescriptions or advice. Please use them as a starting point for discussion. Please also note that these are general notes and, as such, they are not directed at an individual subject. The content of my book *The TDOS Syndrome* is not intended to treat, cure, or be a substitute for proven medical advice, treatments, protocols, or prescription drug therapies. None of these statements has been evaluated by the Food and Drug Administration. It is always recommended to check with your health professional before embarking on any new diet, nutrition, or exercise program.

Foreword

Bernd Lauber, MD

Diplomat of the American Board of Anesthesiology

The content presented in Peter Greenlaw's book, *The TDOS Syndrome*, is, in my view, both visionary and revolutionary. Visionary, because it gives a bird's eye view of some of the most significant issues threatening our individual health and how those issues interact with each other synergistically. This has repercussions for our society's ability to survive into the future. Revolutionary, because it approaches our problems with a new perspective that is completely different from any current recommendations about what it takes to remain healthy.

In the US our standard of living is facing some tough challenges. We are on the threshold of a frightening reality. Our population is aging, as the population bulge of the Baby Boom snakes through the life cycle, with 10,000 Boomers retiring every day. Additionally, with the increasing needs of our aging population, personal and financial support will be needed from subsequent generations who will have to provide for this sector through their contributions. The financial burden is daunting. The difficulty arises due to the discrepancy between the large numbers of Boomers versus the smaller populations of the generations that follow. In addition, we are in a frightening escalation of several significant health trends.

Health-care costs have spiraled out of control. The current dialogue in Washington between both political parties is unhealthy. The rhetoric of a "slowdown" of the rate of rise in health-care costs, as projected by the supporters of the Affordable Care Act, completely ignores the fact that, as a population, some of the toughest battles with regard to our health as a nation have only recently begun to be understood.

Our health-care system is focused on treating disease once it manifests. This increases treatment costs. We treat osteoporosis or high blood pressure once they develop. We treat type 2 diabetes with oral medications and only marginally approach "real" lifestyle, diet, and exercise changes. We treat high cholesterol with expensive and not entirely risk-free statin drugs. We address sleep apnea with uncomfortable oxygen masks or surgery. We perform expensive and risky surgeries on our morbidly obese patients.

These examples point to how medicine is practiced in the United States today; it is predominantly reactive. That is, we wait for disease to manifest and then we intervene with pharmaceuticals, surgery, or other procedures. While necessary and not entirely avoidable, it is time that we begin to approach our health, or lack thereof, in a much more proactive, pre-emptive, personal, and individual manner.

Peter Greenlaw's book highlights four co-factors that, together, are magnifying the downward spiral of our health. The culprits are toxins, nutritional deficiency, overweight, and stress: The TDOS Syndrome.

Toxins: Our bodies face an increasing toxic burden of harmful chemicals that assault us everywhere—in the air we breathe, the water we drink, and the food we consume. We are regularly exposed to a chemical cocktail of roughly 80,000 substances. Only a few have ever been tested regarding their long-term effects on human health. Our understanding of their interactions with our bodies is at best incomplete. A flurry of information is coming to light about the toxicity of some of these chemicals. The picture it paints is potentially grim, a frightening canvas that depicts the future of the human species.

Chemicals like Bisphenol A and the commonly used weed killer Glyphosate, which finds extensive use in modern agricultural practices, are potent endocrine disruptors. The chemicals affect our endocrine system, which functions in close concert with our reproductive system, affecting the hormonal systems and the fertility of our adult population. What is even more frightening is that they can and will have an influence on the immature, developing systems of our children at an early age, when their bodies are most prone to programming errors that will affect them for the rest of their lives. These toxic chemicals potentially threaten our ability to procreate. Such an impact imperils the survival of the human species on this planet.

Nutritional Deficiency: The standard nutritional recommendations from physicians, dieticians, clinical nutritionists, and other health professionals are: consume a well-balanced, diversified diet of carbohydrates, proteins, and fats, with focus on fruits and vegetables and healthy fats and oils. They recommend limiting red meats, processed foods, and simple sugars. It's challenging to maintain a healthy diet. Meanwhile we are bombarded by well-intended advice, along with sales pitches and distorted opinions and recommendations from special interest groups in our industrialized food production system.

The industrial food industry mass-produces cheap food with a long shelf life to feed an ever-growing global population. In my opinion, the quality of the foods we consume has steadily declined. Little nutrition remains. After reading the following pages in *The TDOS Syndrome*, you will have a better understanding of this discrepancy.

The paradox: We are a nation that is overfed but sadly undernourished. As the author poignantly observes, "Food will never be enough by itself." This sentiment certainly rings true for me in my own study of this topic. We need to look at food as not only providing us with needed macronutrients—carbohydrates, fats, and proteins—and thus the calories (just like gasoline that keeps the engine running) but also in terms of the overall content of micronutrients.

Micronutrients are the crucial vitamins, trace minerals, phytonutrients, enzymes, and so on. Today we see the steep decline in micronutrients in our raw food, a century in the making. The unknowing consumer is not informed about the lack of nutrients in our food.

The food companies obfuscate these facts and blur the truth to maintain the status quo.

An interesting study published in 2009 illustrates this point. The incidence of multiple micronutrient deficiencies is more prevalent in overweight and obese adults, as well as children. In other words, those dietary habits that lead to excess weight gain also predispose the individual to have nutrient deficiencies! When you add a calorie-reduction diet on top of the micronutrient deficiency and overall nutritional deficiency of raw food products, it is not surprising that typical diets fail. Even focusing on the so-called healthy foods isn't sufficient. Nutrients are depleted even there. Our bodies simply cannot sustain functioning with a further nutrient shortage.

Another interesting recent study points to a link between weight-loss diets and an actual increase in blood levels of toxins and also between diabetes and blood levels of toxins. This supports the author's hypothesis that toxicity, nutrient deficiencies, and being overweight are directly interlinked.

Overweight: This poses another huge threat to our society as a whole. As a population, we are growing. I mean that in the literal sense. The percentage of extremely overweight people is at an all-time high. Our children and even our babies are fatter and in worse physical shape than they have ever been.

Where, on the continuum from overweight to obesity, do long-term ill-health effects begin? While it depends on the individual, there is no question that financially devastating chronic diseases appear in those suffering from excess weight problems at a higher incidence.

Some of the common problems that I see nearly every day in my medical practice include heart disease, high blood pressure, diabetes, gastrointestinal reflux, sleep apnea, cancer, back pain and injuries, inflammatory diseases, and more. These cause tremendous personal hardships for the individuals but also place a huge financial burden on our country.

It will, in my opinion, become absolutely unsustainable and threaten to bankrupt our nation. Current estimates project that the annual expenditures associated with obesity-related diseases will grow from a current $150–170 billion to a projected $500 billion or more by the year 2030!

These are annual costs with the potential to increase exponentially, adding to our national debt. We can try to rein in our costs as much as we want through legislation. Until we get serious about the underlying root cause of these expenses (and our health), we will fail miserably, both as individuals and as a society.

Stress: A favorite buzzword, stress forces us to run from crisis to crisis and to put out one fire after another with little reprieve for refueling and replenishing in between. We all know stress is bad and that we need to avoid it as much as possible. That is easier said than done. While we may have some degree of control over external causes of stress, most of us don't understand what stress does internally. Many have heard about the links to heart disease, high blood pressure, and anxiety. Many people overeat because of stress. The problem runs much deeper than that.

The factors described above, along with the constant assault of chronic excess stress, which puts our body in a constant defensive and repair mode, creates a vicious vortex of self-perpetuating processes that insidiously accelerate our aging process and make us sicker faster.

We are bombarded with advice on lifestyle, diet, and exercise. Yet, despite all of this information available to us, the sad truth is that most of us will falter and succumb along the road. Mr. Greenlaw has a wonderful ability to break down the problems with a novel perspective and then to reassemble them, showing the interconnections that make sense out of the bigger picture.

In his next book, *The TDOS Solutions*, Greenlaw and his coauthors provide solutions that are both systematic as well as realistically attainable by each and every one of us. The choice of whether to continue with the status quo, or not, is up to us. The government, well intended as it may be, and our current health-care system, are ill equipped to affect changes at the scale called for.

I challenge you to read the information contained in these two books, to really understand the magnitude of the problem. Reading first about the syndrome and then about the solutions protocol, you will be amazed at the transformation that you are about to experience.

It's Not Too Late for You to Change

For most people, a "do-over" in life is a rare opportunity. If you are fortunate enough to receive a chance at a do-over, I suggest you take it. I am one of the lucky ones who got to hit the reset button before it was too late for my family and me.

If you are reading this book, you have that incredible chance for making a big change to improve your quality of life—before it becomes too late.

My own story is instructive. More than a decade ago, I found myself sitting in my doctor's office, awaiting my yearly physical results. The look on the doctor's face told me something was terribly wrong.

He said, "Peter, your lab results prompt me to warn you that if you do not do something radically different starting today, when you walk out of here, you will probably never meet your grandchildren. Your heart attack risk on a scale of 1 to 100 is at 85, and you do not want to go higher. My stern recommendation is severe diet restriction, aggressive exercise, and statin drugs. You have to get on this right away."

When he proposed diet and exercise, *I figured I can lick this*, no problem. You see, I had been on the University of Colorado ski team and at one point had trained at a world-class level. So I thought that if I attacked this problem by exercising rigorously, eating like a rabbit, and taking my medications, somehow my health and prospects for a long life would return to normal.

At the end of two months trying this regimen, I was shocked to discover that I had lost only eight pounds. Even more disturbing to me was the realization that despite having increased my amount of statin drugs by 500 percent, my risk factor for an early death had barely been reduced. Needless to say, I was shaken and scared.

What had gone wrong? Why had mainstream medical advice and a traditional strategy for renewing and maintaining health so utterly failed me?

Then a sort of miracle happened. A friend of mine, Jim, introduced me to a do-over, a second chance, and I will forever be indebted to him. At the time, what he suggested was a new nutritional approach, but I embraced it. You will learn more about my experience with it later. Today, I truly believe it is the reason why I lived to meet my granddaughters, Evelyn and Gwyneth, and my grandson, Barrett.

In a matter of days after adopting this new health strategy, I lost as much weight as I had in two months using the old philosophy of diet, exercise, and medications. I will never forget when, only a few days into the new protocol, I looked down and thought my scale was broken. I said to myself, *if this is real, it's going to change the world.*

I wound up losing more than 30 pounds.

Even better news was yet to come. I went back to see my doctor after two months of being on this revolutionary new nutritional approach, and when he came in to the room with my test results, he said, "I am sorry, we have to run the tests again."

"Why?" I asked.

"Because, according to these results, your heart attack risk has gone from 85 to 15," he said, sounding incredulous. "I want to repeat the tests to make sure there's no mistake in the analysis. By the way, how much of the statin drugs are you taking?"

"I have not taken statins in two months," I replied. "I simply overhauled my diet."

My doctor stared back at me in disbelief. "Okay, keep doing what you're doing and come back in two months."

It turned out that the results of my diagnostic tests were accurate. A dramatic transformation in my health was underway.

But why did that happen, and how? This set in motion a comprehensive research and discovery process, enabling me to see how a nutritional approach held the potential to create a pivotal change in human health.

MY SEARCH FOR ANSWERS

In the spirit of full disclosure, I am not a trained biologist, nutritionist, or scientist; nor am I a medical doctor. I stumbled into my role as a health advocate by being an investigator of health sciences—as a layman scientist, if you will—while trying to improve my own health. Over a period of thirteen years, I read several hundred books and conversed for countless hours with medical experts, concerning their respective findings. I was relentless in seeking answers to my health questions. Though I found that the specialists—all leaders in diverse areas of health—had amassed the best information available, most had failed to see the bigger picture. It was going to take an outsider to put all the pieces together, which is the task I assigned myself.

When I received my blood work results, after ten weeks of the natural detox protocol I had been on, thanks to Jim, those heartening results combined with my huge weight loss were my first realization that something had occurred to me that had profound implications.

Another pivotal moment arrived when I read the book *Our Toxic World: A Wakeup Call* by Dr. Doris Rapp, an environmental medicine specialist, who was a past President of the American Academy of Environmental Medicine. Her pioneering book published in 2003 documented some of the health effects of exposure to chemicals in products. She had been a Clinical Professor of Pediatrics at the State University of New York. Dr. Rapp is also a board-certified environmental medical specialist, pediatric allergist, and homeopath. She certainly knew what she was talking about concerning human health and our environment.

She revealed how toxins were having a major impact on childhood allergies, and she was one of the first to describe how toxins in the environment were doing more harmful things to us than medicine or science had yet discovered or fully acknowledged.

Before meeting her, I believed that if you simply lost weight, you became healthier. I knew nothing about the role of toxins. After reading her book, I was so taken with her premise that I tracked her down and spent four days with her in Scottsdale, Arizona, learning everything I could about her theories. There were very few people talking or writing in depth about this subject at that time, beyond her.

Face time with someone is irreplaceable, and so it was with her. She conveyed to me how toxins were a ticking time bomb, a major health problem, and no one had yet comprehended the bigger picture. She liked the fact that I had this fascination with the subject, a curiosity to learn, and that I possessed an enthusiasm to inform others. She encouraged me to bring this message to the world, because it would impact our children.

The task of assembling the evidence, and disseminating it, seemed monumental. It felt a bit intimidating to take on such a huge project. But Dr. Rapp opened my eyes to an entire hidden reality, and I began developing this growing curiosity and determination to learn more.

Why are so few people talking to each other or their doctors about this? I kept asking myself, even though I knew one reason was because there had been so few scientific studies on toxins accumulating in humans and their health implications. Armed with some of the information that I had collected, I started speaking to others about detoxification and weight loss. My first public talk, in March 2004, was at a library in Denver. My presentation was titled "Toxicity in America." Only a few people attended, most of them family members. Keep in mind that in those early days we thought the whole magic was weight loss, as a result of the natural detox I had discovered. I kept witnessing people lose huge amounts of weight from the detox regimen I was using.

The concept is that the body's natural detoxification process is dependent on receiving key nutrients. If these nutrients are not received, the process does not function properly, and this increases stress on the body. The increased stress causes accumulation of fat that leads to overweight. This in turn leads to more stress, more toxic burden, and hampers the body's ability to absorb the necessary nutrients. Thus, Toxicity, Deficiency, Overweight, and Stress, interact with each other in a tightening spiral, which we call TDOS Syndrome.

Meanwhile, more of the science was gradually emerging.

A 2005 laboratory study on the umbilical cord blood taken from ten babies, conducted by the Environmental Working Group, was a real wake-up call for anyone concerned with the future of human health. Of 287 industrial chemicals (such as stain and oil repellants from fast food packaging) that scientists for the group detected in that umbilical cord blood, 180 of the chemicals were known to cause cancer, 217 were toxic to the brain and nervous system, and 208 caused birth defects or abnormal development.

This study and related research gave rise to the term "body burden," referring to the load of toxins the average human body absorbs in a normal lifetime, and winds up storing in fat tissue, as if the body were an industrial pharmacy. Bill Moyers of the Public Broadcasting System had been tested for his body burden of chemicals at Mount Sinai Hospital in New York City. The results came back positive for 84 of the 154 chemicals for which he was tested, including 31 different types of PCBs, 13 different dioxins, and pesticides, such as DDT. That produced a brief flurry of publicity.

Next, an investigative journalist wrote a book, *The Hundred Year Lie: How Food and Medicine are Destroying Your Health*, released during the summer of 2006 by a major publisher. The book revealed for the first time the health impacts of toxic synergies, individual toxins from industrial products that interact with each other and once inside the body intensify their harmful effects.

A few months later in October 2006, *National Geographic* published a detailed article titled "The Pollution Within," in which the writer became "journalist as guinea pig," and had his blood and urine tested for toxins at Mount Sinai Hospital. Traces of hundreds of toxic chemicals were found in his body, everything from flame-retardants to mercury. Many were endocrine system disrupters.

Another important connection for me also emerged in 2006 when two scientists at the University of California, Irvine, in the Department of Developmental and Cell Biology, published two studies coining the term "obesogens" to refer to a new mode of action they had discovered for endocrine system disrupting chemicals—triggering obesity in humans. Certain chemicals alter our hormones and affect fat cells, contributing to weight gain and making it more difficult to lose weight. Not only that, subsequent research would detail how these chemicals can affect fetuses in the womb, making obesity hereditary.

Pieces of the puzzle were fast coming together. (You will find much more on all of these revelations and their interconnections later in this book.)

All of these findings should have been treated at the time as health-shaking developments, trumpeted to the public with the urgency and attention of a loud, marching band. Yet we heard next to nothing about these hidden accumulating threats to our well-being and future as a species.

At this point, I didn't yet grasp that toxins were running wild inside of us partly because we didn't have the nutrients in our body to help eliminate them. Our poor diets caused these nutrient deficiencies. I learned about this connection in a book by an environmental medicine physician, Sherry A. Rogers. *Detoxify or Die* discussed the importance of glutathione as a toxin scavenger. The importance she placed on this nutrient grabbed my attention. Rogers is board certified by the American Board of Family Practice and the American Board of Environmental Medicine, and she is a Fellow of the American College of Allergy, Asthma & Immunology and a Fellow of the American College of Nutrition, so she certainly had the credentials to be writing authoritatively about the connections between toxins, nutrients, and detoxification.

Another influential read for me was *The Cortisol Connection* by Shawn Talbott, a PhD nutritionist in sports medicine. That book proved to be another turning point, an informational catalyst that prompted me to look at stress, and its implications, in a broader way. Chronic release of cortisol, the stress hormone, shuts down the immune system, reduces bone density, shrinks our brain, and spikes insulin so the body stores more fat. Research revealed that even introducing the thought of going on a diet increased cortisol levels in test subjects.

DISCOVERING THE TDOS SYNDROME®

My final big epiphany, one of those "Eureka" moments that tied together everything I had learned, occurred as I was writing a book about aging. Stanford Medical School had released findings that stress was a contributing factor to early death. I was sitting at my desk, typing some sentences about how stress speeds up our aging process, when it hit me. Stress was a major contributor to being overweight, and being overweight was connected to nutrient deficiencies, which was connected to the absorption of toxins in a vicious cycle of four co-factors.

"Oh, my gosh!" I exclaimed. "It all fits."

To be sure of the significance of what I detected, I needed the outside opinion of a medical authority, so I immediately looked up a physician, Nicholas Messina, who I had known for several years. He was someone I respected as a researcher because he had worked on numerous major drug trials for pharmaceutical companies, developing new drugs.

I phoned him and said, "listen, doc, give me your feedback. I think I've made a major discovery."

After describing my theory and some of the findings behind it, he said, "That is intriguing. I think this could represent a syndrome. A syndrome is a group of signs and symptoms that occur together and characterize a particular abnormality or condition. In this case Toxicity, Deficiency, Overweight and Stress all connect and lead to accelerated cellular aging. You should be able to patent this term."

The four co-factors acting together as a synergy did resemble a syndrome, and from my conversation with Dr. Messina, TDOS Syndrome was born as a term and a title:

- T for toxins
- D for nutrient deficiencies
- O for overweight
- S for stress

When I asked Dr. Messina to collaborate on a book with me about these findings and the syndrome, he accepted.

MY BROTHER'S URGENT PLEA

Along the way, as my research journey unfolded, several people I highly respected encouraged me to persevere and continue digging. They sensed that I was on to something important, which was the validation I needed. My younger brother Patrick became one of these sources of inspiration.

Patrick had been a prominent television news anchor on CNN and other broadcast stations throughout his 25-year career as a public figure. In 2011 Patrick had what we thought were just chronic back pains. I finally convinced him to see an orthopedic doctor for an MRI.

It was a beautiful Colorado Monday morning with a brilliant blue sky and bright sun, as I waited in the reception area while Patrick met with the physician. A nurse came to tell me that Patrick needed to see me. When I opened the door and saw Patrick, a 6´5˝ man, doubled over crying, I immediately knew something was horribly wrong. He got up, hugged me, and said the doctor had found a massive tumor on his kidney.

The rest of that day is a blur. We learned from an oncologist that Patrick had a stage IV malignant tumor—the size of a baseball—wrapped around his spine, and if he did not have immediate surgery, it would paralyze him.

Patrick had surgery four days later and immediately began oral chemotherapy. His surgery lasted more than eight hours, and the doctors removed the bulk of the tumor. Unfortunately, he continued to deteriorate, despite the surgery and medical treatments. He was hospitalized several more times from side effects of his chemotherapy treatments, and eventually he underwent radiation therapy as well.

The last night I visited with Patrick in the hospital, it was obvious he wasn't going to receive a second chance. Although he was valiantly fighting to stay alive, there would be no do-over. Only eight short months after the tumor was discovered, we were told there was nothing more that medical specialists could do for him.

Patrick and I spent this night talking about our lives, our gratefulness for everything we had, and how much we wished we could have do-overs regarding so many things in life. We laughed and cried as brothers in a way that we never had before.

Patrick said several times, "I can't believe I'm going to die."

He cried deeply, and the emotive force of it broke my heart. I had just told him that I would cancel my next week's speaking tour to spend more time with him when the most prophetic words came out of his mouth.

He stunned me by saying, "Peter, what you're working on is a news story, a really big story. I don't want you sitting around here watching me die. I want you to go out and tell the world what you have discovered. It's your job to make the world aware of what's happening and what's possible. Because, if there is one person who can have a second chance before it's too late for them, do it for me."

I had great respect for my brother and his encouragement inspired me to summon the dogged determination that I needed to carry on. Reluctantly, I left him and flew out to speak that Monday morning, the same day they transferred Patrick back to his home for hospice care.

On Friday night, 30 minutes before I was scheduled to speak in Washington, D.C., I received a call from Patrick's wife, Debra. She said, "Peter, talk to Patrick. He is in terrible pain. Tell him to stop fighting."

Although I wasn't even sure he would understand me because of the morphine he was taking, I managed to tell him through my tears, "Patrick let go. It's okay. Debra and your daughter, Brittany, will be okay. You have suffered enough."

Debra thanked me, and I went on stage to speak at 7:00 p.m.

Unbeknownst to me, while I was on that stage, my wonderful younger brother Patrick passed away.

Telling this story is still extremely emotional and painful for me. There are some nights when I still break down in tears when I talk about Patrick. Hopefully, you can sense the depth of my passion and my driving need to spread this message. If I had known what I now have come to understand, maybe, just maybe, that knowledge could have given Patrick a second chance.

Unlike my brother Patrick, it may not be too late for you.

Yes, you may really get a second chance, a do-over, or a reset.

If you have loved ones who have become health statistics, and you have seen firsthand their suffering from the onslaught of systemic health failures, then you know how that experience can smother you into a shocked silence, feeling helplessness and despair. Or the experience can change you and inflame you with a burning passion to launch your own health crusade, so the agony of disease isn't visited upon another single human being.

As you probably sense by now, I emerged from these wrenching experiences setting an intention to change the world.

A BRIGHTER HEALTH FUTURE

Along with some other collaborators Dr. Messina and I gathered along the way, the information in this book is the culmination of a two-part journey of discovery. In *The TDOS Syndrome* we will explain the TDOS problem and provide evidence for this syndrome, which is ruining the health of millions of people. In our next book we will offer the TDOS Solutions, in which we present our preventive and regenerative solutions to the unprecedented health problems we have identified that humankind now urgently faces.

We encourage you to weigh the evidence with an open mind.

If you're a little skeptical right now, that's okay. At first I too was a skeptic. But that attitude gradually dissolved as the puzzle pieces came together and I discovered the growing and ominous picture of our future.

Many people, particularly those whose incomes rely on maintaining the status quo when it comes to our deteriorating health status, may react negatively when confronted with such harsh doses of reality. That is to be expected. It's how our health system has worked—and failed—for far too long, and that attitude and situation must change.

My coauthors and I don't claim to cure any disease, nor is TDOS Syndrome itself a disease. Our intent is to raise your awareness, to give you options, and most of all to make you *think*. We hope you can come to your own conclusions. We simply want you to see how these new discoveries may be something you want to incorporate in creating a healthier lifestyle for yourself and, equally important, for the people you love and care about.

Acknowledgments

To my fabulous literary agent, Bill Gladstone, of Waterside Productions for so believing in *The TDOS Syndrome.*

Also a huge thanks to Kenzi Sugihara of SelectBooks for a huge leap of faith in taking us on.

With sincere gratitude for the tireless consulting on this book by the amazing author, Randall Fitzgerald.

I want to thank Bill Andrews, PhD, in population genetics and molecular biology, whom I call, simply, Einstein. Bill taught me Telomere science and allowed me access to his amazing company, Sierra Sciences, which is located in Reno, Nevada.

Additionally, I thank Dr. Dennis Harper (Coauthor of *Why Diets are Failing US*) for his amazing guidance to a novice in the world of medicine and nutritional science.

My special thanks to Dr. Bernd Lauber for his contribution to my research and to this book.

Next, a big thanks to my business partner, Scott, who hung in there with me even when he thought perhaps I would never finish my book.

A special thanks to Kirk Metz, who was instrumental in helping me stay on track with my research. He is one of the greatest personal development trainers I have ever met.

Thank you to Doug Freel, my amazing director and coproducer for having the vision and confidence to create our upcoming TV show called *The Greenlaw Report*™.

A huge thanks to my oldest son, Drew Greenlaw, graduate of the University of Colorado School of Journalism. His fearless and tireless efforts turned my ramblings into this book.

I thank Nicholas Messina, MD, my collaborator and coauthor, for lending credibility to this book with his medical expertise and great insights. He has been an amazing mentor.

The greatest thanks to my home team, my youngest son and loving wife, Sarah. She has always believed in me. Thank you to Colin for his cheerleading and constant belief in me.

Introduction

A Perfect Health Storm

Maybe you've seen or heard about the movie *The Perfect Storm*, featuring George Clooney. This film title is based on real weather terminology related to an event that occurred in 1991 along the East Coast of the United States. A ridge of high pressure extended from the Appalachian Mountains northeastward to Greenland. This cold air and high pressure over eastern Canada blocked the warm moist air from the south. This interaction spawned an "extra-tropical low" and an associated massive ocean-centered cyclone that gathered up the warm, humid remnants of Hurricane Grace. With the cold and dry high-pressure system meeting the warm, damp, low pressure, the destructive force of the perfect storm magnified to tragic proportions. It caused death and massive damage, all without even making landfall.

Now, imagine what it might look like if *four* such storm centers converged at the same time. The synergy (all four interacting together) of that convergence would be devastating, to an extent unparalleled in recorded history. That type of synergy is occurring right now, in the realm of human health, with four co-factors having combined to wreak havoc on an unsuspecting public. The TDOS Syndrome is the biggest—and most under the radar superstorm in the history of human health and wellness. And almost no one is aware of it, or doing anything about it. The rates of cancer, cardiovascular disease, diabetes, Alzheimer's disease, and more are increasing exponentially due to the effects of the TDOS Syndrome. It even affects our very ability to procreate.

In this book we'll take a careful look at each of the four co-factors—toxicity, nutritional deficiency, overweight, and stress—and explain why they are harmful both individually and collectively. We hope to empower you with the information you need to make better health choices in the future.

A DANGEROUS SYNERGY

Synergy is one of the governing principles of nature. We see it or feel it at work everywhere in our lives, yet we rarely recognize the phenomenon. Think of it as two or more of anything—chemicals, ingredients, climate patterns, and so on—interacting to produce effects much more powerful than any one of them can generate on its own.

There are both positive and negative (toxic) synergies. For example, positive synergy is when the various nutrients (minerals, phytochemicals, and fiber) in an apple interact once ingested to promote a range of health benefits, such as protection from cardiovascular disease. Negative, toxic synergies can include various pesticides combining in the human body to kill brain cells, resulting in neurological disorders such as Alzheimer's disease.

A toxin that is present in extremely minute quantities, in the parts per billion, can be harmless on its own when a human being is exposed to it. Yet, when this toxin interacts with other seemingly harmless toxins in relatively small amounts, together they can magnify their effects and become a roaring beast of health disruption and destruction.

For our purposes in this book, synergy refers to both the interactions between the four co-factors of TDOS (Toxins, Deficiency in nutrients, Over-weight, and Stress), as well as interactions within each of the co-factors, such as the countless toxic chemical synergies that trigger health problems.

Our Health Devastation by the Numbers

To begin comprehending the visible manifestations of how the TDOS Syndrome synergy is wreaking havoc, we only need to begin with some of the alarming health casualty figures:

Cancer: In 1990 one in fifteen US women were diagnosed with breast cancer. It is now one in eight. If this trend continues, the American Cancer Society estimates that one in three women will develop breast cancer in the next decade.[1]

For all types of cancer, a man's lifetime chance of developing an invasive cancer is one in two; for women, the lifetime chance is one in three. Over the past decade, diagnosed cases of these cancers increased substantially: kidney, liver, thyroid, esophageal, testicular, melanoma. Leukemia, brain cancer, and childhood cancers in general increased more than 20 percent since the 1970s.[2]

One major big reason given for the explosion in cancer cases was identified in 2010 by the President's Cancer Panel: *human absorption of chemical toxins in the environment.*[3]

Cardiovascular Disease: This is an entire category of circulatory problems, including heart attacks, strokes, and the circulatory disease itself known as cardiovascular disease. Between 1990 and 2013 global deaths due to this disease increased by 41 percent, reaching nearly 18 million people annually.[4]

Obesity and Overweight: By comparing the body mass index of nearly 20 million adult men and women from nearly 200 countries, compiled from 1975 to 2014, British scientists determined in 2016 that *obesity in men has tripled and obesity in women has more than doubled* over three decades. The highest obesity rates were in the US and China.[5]

Diabetes: Diagnosed cases of diabetes worldwide nearly *quadrupled from 1980 to 2014*, according to the World Health Organization, affecting more than 400 million people. That means nearly 10 percent of all adults on the planet now have this deadly killer disease of high blood sugar levels, which are primarily the type 2, rather than type 1 diabetes.[6]

Alzheimer's Disease: This neurological degeneration affects more than five million Americans each year. Based on current case growth, by the year 2050 the number of people with Alzheimer's is expected to triple, according to the Alzheimer's Association. During the past decade alone, deaths from this disease rose by 71 percent, which translates into more than 700,000 deaths a year.[7]

Parkinson's Disease: While in 2005 there were 4.1 million people with this neurological disease, by the year 2040 that number will more than double, reported the Parkinson's Disease Foundation. It is theorized that genetic predisposition "loads the gun," and that environmental influences "pull the trigger" to bring about the disease. Those environmental influences have been identified as including exposure to a variety of pesticides, solvents such as TCE, and PCBs (polychlorinated biphenyls).[8]

Infertility and Pregnancy Difficulties: Over three decades the numbers of couples reporting infertility, or difficulty in conceiving and maintaining a pregnancy, increased dramatically. Since 1982 at least 40 percent more women have had these problems, while difficulties in younger women, ages 18 to 25, nearly doubled in the same period.[9]

Asthma: In only fifteen years, from 1980 to 1995, diagnosed cases of asthma doubled. By 2009 an estimated one in twelve people in the US, mostly young people, had asthma and its symptoms.[10]

Learning and Developmental Disabilities: If we add together attention deficit hyperactivity disorder and autism, along with diagnosed learning and developmental disabilities, one in six US children are affected. Autism diagnoses alone have seen a 300 percent increase in the US since 1997.[11]

Fatty Liver Disease: Non-alcoholic fatty liver disease affects nearly 10 percent of all children in the US, according to the American Liver Foundation. Perhaps most alarming is that a few decades ago this disease had never before been seen in children. It is caused by genetic background and environmental triggers that combine to create fat accumulation in the liver.[12]

Stress (Chronic): Though comparative annual statistics are unavailable, the most recent surveys of US adults have found that 77 percent report "regularly experiencing physical symptoms caused by stress," and 73 percent report "regularly experiencing psychological symptoms caused by stress." Half of everyone surveyed also reported that their stress levels increased over the previous five years.[13]

All of the above diseases and ailments have the following two statements in common:

1. Statistics reveal that all have been on the increase since the 1950s, after the explosion in the numbers of chemicals being manufactured following World War II.

2. All have some documented or theorized connection to toxins as causative agents responsible for these jumps in diagnosed cases.

THE PIECES OF A HEALTH PUZZLE

During my research, a realization emerged that health and wellness beliefs have been formed based on old truths that are no longer accurate. Many of our health and wellness assumptions—what we think we know about eating, food, calories, and diets, about toxins and nutritional deficiency, about weight management and stress—are fundamentally wrong.

Nothing demonstrates the prevailing flawed premises and health assumptions more than the discovery of a TDOS Syndrome. The four co-factors of TDOS, the four deadly horsemen of the health apocalypse, are:

Toxicity

Deficiency (nutritional deficiency)

Overweight

Stress

TDOS Syndrome is the interconnectivity of four individual co-factors that have united to play a large role not only in sabotaging the body's natural ability to function optimally but also in preventing the body from losing weight. When these four co-factors combine, it sets off a perfect storm in the body, preventing the body from working as efficiently as it should. While each factor alone weakens our health, together they threaten it so much more powerfully that our future as a species is endangered.

Since TDOS Syndrome is a collaborative problem, we can look at it two ways. First, we can examine how each co-factor builds on the others and its power to magnify our collective health problems. Second, we can pick apart each co-factor as it wreaks havoc individually and see the specific effects of each one.

Toxicity

The first of the four co-factors, *toxicity* plays a significant role in dieting and weight loss. The body is in a state of evolution. For centuries humans weren't bombarded with the toxic soup that we now swim through every day. The air was pure. Only people dealing with toxic chemicals in science labs or soldiers battling in chemical warfare areas used gas masks or breathing filters. People would have looked at you like you had two heads if you walked down the street with an air filter mask on during a heavy pollution day. People could drink from a fresh water stream, and kids drank straight from the hose in the backyard

on a hot summer day. Water supplies didn't need to go through puri-
fication stations to remove sewage, chemicals, and even pharmaceuticals. There was also no need to "enhance" water supplies with fluoride
or other minerals. Our food supplies weren't riddled with herbicides
and pesticides. Animals weren't pumped full of growth hormones and
there was no need to re-enhance foods with vitamins and minerals
that are now missing from our food supplies. Because of this onslaught
of toxicity, the human body has created its own toxins called "obesogens." The main problem regarding weight loss is that the body
refuses to release excess weight because to do so is a direct threat to
poisoning the body with these toxins.

Deficiency

Nutritional *deficiency* plays a huge role on its own as discussed in
the book but also as a co-factor. When the body does not receive optimal nutrition, it won't function at the highest level. As we already
know, our food supplies no longer have sufficient levels of the vitamins and minerals needed for the body to operate normally. Most diet
approaches include some type of caloric restriction, but when calories are cut, the amount of nutrition is also drastically diminished,
meaning the body receives less of what it needs to function properly.
The body needs proper proportions of protein, carbohydrates, and fats,
as well as vitamins and minerals. For example, if you start an exercise program, the body needs protein to help with both building muscle and recovery. When the body is riddled with toxicity, it makes it
harder for the body to process any nutrition, and when there is a lack
of nutrition to begin with, every problem becomes magnified. Keep
in mind that the one constant throughout the last half-century is that
the nutritional content of our food continues to decrease. Combine that
nutritional decrease with diets high in processed foods, fat, and sugar,
and you have the perfect recipe for an unhealthy state in the body—a
body that is out of balance.

Overweight

If you are *overweight* or obese or thin, there is a good chance that your body is dealing with a certain degree of toxic burden. Yes, the body holds excess fat due to poor nutrition, bad eating habits, and a lack of exercise. But as you are beginning to see, it is no longer as easy to lose weight by simply dieting and exercising. If the body is flooded with toxins, weight loss becomes almost impossible due to the fact that the excess fat is protecting the body from itself. If the surplus of fat is released without some kind of nutritional fasting program, it is possible that it could flood the body with toxicity, causing any number of problems and potentially making that individual sick. When adding overweight to both toxicity and deficiency, we begin to really see how each co-factor plays individual roles as well as their combined effects, and it starts to look like it is virtually impossible to get healthy and lose weight. When it comes to a lifestyle change in order to lose weight, the first step most people consider is a diet.

Yet going on a typical "diet" these days almost guarantees a weight gain in the long run. If this is your story, you should ask yourself two questions: Why am I dieting and how am I dieting? Usually, the simple answer to the first question is to lose weight. The second question certainly has a myriad of different answers, ranging from exercise, calorie reduction, medication, and—in some drastic situations—surgery. These techniques are not as effective as they once were. One major reason that dieting no longer works as advertised in the long term is due certainly in part to the impact of the TDOS Syndrome.

Stress

Stress is the last co-factor in the TDOS Syndrome, and most everyone is aware of, or feels, this deadly co-factor. Stress is a killer on its own. People who are otherwise in good health have been decimated by stress. Whether it's from the daily stresses of life or the actual internal stress placed on the body from poor health or being overweight, stress is not to be taken lightly. As we know, external life stresses can raise blood pressure among other things. Excess weight also places a significant amount of stress on the body. It literally "stresses" all of the body's functions from how the heart and lungs operate to adding excess pressure to ankles, knees, and the back. Once again, stress alone is a killer; add it to the other three co-factors, and you have the perfect storm called the TDOS Syndrome.

FROM SYNERGY TO SYNDROME

We have this health problem puzzle, with all of the pieces scattered. Yes, you can find a couple of the pieces, put them together, and ascertain a part of the bigger picture. But it's not until you connect the entire puzzle, seeing that the pieces really do fit, that you begin to learn how to search for the necessary solutions.

The four co-factors are harmful enough on their own, but once I saw the interconnectivity and the interdependency, I understood the multiplier effect. It's a previously unidentified synergy. There are so many angles of connectivity to unravel. To cite one example, it became clear to me that a deficiency in our foods, the absence of important nutrients, allows toxins to run wild inside the human body by depriving the body's detoxification mechanism of what it needs to function properly. In turn, if you are nutritionally deficient, it triggers stress. When stress rises, so does insulin and cortisol. When that occurs, the emergence of obesity and diabetes are not far behind.

The synergy of these four co-factors constitutes the syndrome. No one was talking about the bigger picture of synergy, so I decided to start the conversation. How can we stop laboring under old misconceptions when it comes to our health and wellness, as well as our ability to live healthier, longer? We can start with one word: *conversation*.

THE NEW HEALTH CONVERSATION

Each one of the TDOS co-factors is deadly in its own right. But in their *interaction* with one another, they become insidious and ultimately debilitating. Together, they create a vicious cycle that plays a major role in the acceleration of aging and the undermining of our collective wellness.

The old conversation about health relied mostly on our brilliant doctors and space-age techniques, medical devices, machines, and wonder drugs. The problem here is that this outdated focus is based on the flawed premise of procedural intervention and disease management. We no longer have a Health Care System; we have a Chronic Disease Management System. Procedural intervention is the technique through which doctors first identify a condition and then prescribe the procedure. Although we clearly have the world's most advanced procedural interventions, this is a *defensive* strategy only. It is not a total solution now, nor will it solve our problems in the future.

We may devise more brilliant procedures, but we must also reduce the *need* for their use, as much as possible, through prevention. The resulting preventive interventional technologies and protocols are part of the new conversation we must have about health. To seek new methods, to find potential solutions, and to create a sustainable and patient-centered system for the future, we must accept that the American health-care system, as it currently exists, is broken. Just as alarmingly, it is bankrupting our nation. As my coauthor Dr. Messina points out, "Until it becomes as profitable to change lifestyles as it is to manage disease, our current health-care system will not change course."

Primary care doctors can be the first line of defense in preventive intervention. Yet, these physicians are vanishing. In the next decade, it is predicted that we may be short as many as 125,000 primary care physicians to meet the country's healthcare needs. Adding to the overload, recent health-care reform, by increasing access to this shrinking pool of doctors, could flood the system with more patients, creating a mini-storm within a super-storm . . . and exponentially increasing the disastrous effects that the TDOS Syndrome is set to unleash on the country.

While our cadres of medical specialists are the envy of the world, and our trauma centers are models of critical care, we spend twice what the rest of the industrialized world spends on health care each year. For all that money we spend, we still rank at the bottom of industrialized nations in life expectancy. This raises serious questions about our current health-care model and whether it is sustainable.

It's time to take control of our lives and stop pretending that it's someone else's obligation. We cannot flout common nutritional sense and "make it all better" with a pill for every ill. We are responsible for our own health, such as ensuring that we are fully aware of the elements that make up the TDOS Syndrome—and then actually doing something about them.

Again, it is important to note that the TDOS Syndrome is not a disease. It is a combination of factors that together undermine your potential to have a high quality of life.

To avoid the health consequences that are robbing us of our life expectancies, we must be proactive and involved in our own health care. I offer you this basic truth: The best medicine is no medicine at all. We can and we must take an active role in *preventive interventional strategies*—starting by engaging in the new health conversation, which relies primarily on new preventive interventional technologies.

In our next book, discussing the TDOS solutions, we will offer you a comprehensive, multi-dimensional strategy of preventive interventions. This new health conversation is essential to help halt what may be one of the most destructive "super-storm" forces to hit the health and well-being of humanity.

I do not write this to scare you to death, but rather, to scare you to *life*.

What we are introducing, my coauthors and I, is a new health conversation. For some of you, this conversation will change your life forever, *if you choose to allow it to do so.*

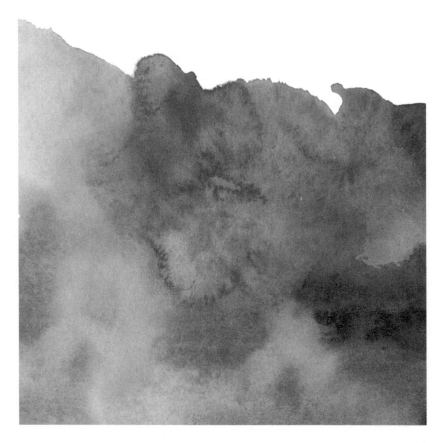

PART ONE

Co-Factor T—**Toxicity**

Co-Factor T—Toxicity

Finding Out What Really Lurks Inside of Us

The US Centers for Disease Control and Prevention (CDC), through its National Center for Health Statistics, has conducted a series of blood and urine tests on thousands of Americans, measuring and monitoring their absorption of chemical toxins, and at what concentrations these chemicals occur in the body. Think of it as an ongoing "Manhattan Project" of public health research.

Four reports have been produced so far: for the years 1999–2000, 2001–2002, 2003–2004, and 2010, with each report summarizing chemical exposure residues (a process called "biomonitoring") as found in about 10,000 people altogether, representing all ages and ethnic backgrounds. These lab tests, which are sophisticated and expensive, provide data on extremely low levels of toxins found in the human body, down to the parts-per-million and parts-per-billion levels of molecule detection.

Each report has expanded the numbers of chemicals that were searched for and ultimately detected in body fluids. In the first report, for instance, dozens of industrial chemicals were on the target list, with each subsequent report adding dozens more chemicals for analysis, until by the fourth report, 212 chemicals had been included.[14]

Unfortunately, many of us contain a large number of these chemicals within our bodies, and they are creating a toxic atmosphere that is seriously damaging our health, partly because many of these toxins build up over time and interact with one another in harmful ways.

They are in the air we breathe, water we drink, food we consume, and personal care products we apply. We are literally drowning in toxins. They are the superbugs of this century, and they are ultimately destroying us.

WHAT IS YOUR "BODY BURDEN"?

Categories of chemicals searched for—and found—in the human test subjects ranged from heavy metals and solvents used in industrial processes to perchlorate (rocket fuel), crop pesticides, insecticides, personal care product chemicals, bisphenol A—found in food can linings—sunblock products like benzophenone, nonstick coating chemicals such as perfluorocarbons, and tricloscan used in antibacterial soaps. All of these chemicals and/or their metabolites (the chemical alteration residue produced by body tissues) were measured according to varying levels in the humans tested. Levels varied based on such factors as exposure frequency and geographic location. Not everyone harbored all of the chemicals in their bodies, but everyone tested was contaminated by many, if not most, of the chemicals.

This chemical contamination is called our "body burden," something every one of us carries. It has become an inescapable reality of modern life that we absorb, and then shelter in our body fat, direct chemical evidence of our industrial evolution as a species.

None of this CDC data, as detailed as it is, gives us information about what concentrations of which chemicals constitute an unsafe health level for us. As the CDC noted in its fourth report: "Research studies, separate from these data, are required to determine which blood or urine levels are safe and which are associated with disease or an adverse effect."[15]

Though it's a seemingly long list of chemicals tested and evaluated in the CDC database so far, it's only a mere fraction (less than 1 percent) of the more than 80,000 synthetic chemicals in common use throughout this country and the world being absorbed by human and animal bodies. If the CDC were to truly undertake testing for the presence of all these more than 80,000 chemicals in the human body, it would be a "Manhattan Project" of complexity and proportions exceeding the building of the first atomic bomb.

Chemical companies claim that low dose exposure to individual chemicals is harmless. But that isn't necessarily true. "A growing body of literature links low dose chemical exposure to a broad range of health effects," noted the Environmental Working Group's scientists, in a report on our body burden. One example is the plasticizer bisphenol A, used in food can linings and plastic water bottles. It can have "health effects with adverse outcomes ranging from altered male reproductive organs and aggressive behavior, to abnormal mammary gland growth, and early puberty."[16]

In any expanded CDC comprehensive testing program, we would also have to consider the additive and synergistic effects of all these chemicals interacting with each other in the human body.

Each of these chemicals acting, on its own, is a potential toxic problem for human health. But multiple chemicals acting together presents a mind-numbing research challenge for the CDC, for the chemical industry, and any independent research team that would attempt to undertake this challenge. There would literally be hundreds of thousands of combinations of chemicals and their synergistic interactions to measure and evaluate for toxicity and their impacts on human health. Now you begin to sense the dimensions of the rather daunting conundrum that confronts us.

We know that each of us carries around a body burden of hundreds, if not thousands, of synthetic chemicals. The exact number is unknown and perhaps, given the current analytical limitations of science, that number is unknowable. Even before birth, we absorb and inherit chemicals directly from our mothers, based on their exposure. We still don't have a clear idea of how much contamination is occurring in the womb, and the extent to which these chemical contaminants linger in us throughout life, wreaking health havoc.

One more thing to keep in mind: Since the US Congress passed the Toxic Substances Control Act in 1976, only about 2 percent of the more than 80,000 chemicals in common use have been tested for their individual impacts on human health. Fewer still have been tested for their "additive" or "synergistic" effects in combination with each other.[17]

Scientific research on the effects of these chemicals inside of us continues to emerge, mostly from independent university and environmental organization testing labs, but only as a slow drip of findings, due to limited financial resources. This chapter will present some of these important findings.

Let's take a deeper dive into how we absorb toxins and how they act as the train engine hooked to, and pulling, the other three TDOS Syndrome co-factors: nutrient deficiencies, overweight, and stress.

WHAT DOES TOXIC REALLY MEAN?

Never lose sight of the fact that humanity is under siege by a ubiquitous, unseen, misunderstood ghost in the form of toxins and manmade toxicants. Toxins are anything in our environment with the potential to negatively affect the health and function of the human body. They enter our bodies through the air we breathe, the water we drink, the food we eat, and even the things we touch, often without our even being aware of it. Many are easily absorbed through the skin, making us particularly susceptible, especially when you consider the numerous products we use on our skin from deodorant to moisturizer to facial cleansers and soaps. Even many sunscreens, designed to protect our skin from harmful rays, contain numerous toxic substances.

"The creation and widespread contamination by man-made, syn-thetic chemicals in the late twentieth century has resulted in every region of the planet being assaulted with a dangerous cocktail of known health-damaging toxins. But how toxic are we?" asked physician and toxins expert, Paula Baillie Hamilton, in her book *Toxic Overload*. We already know the sad state of affairs when it comes to toxicity in the land, the air, and even the sea. But the overriding problem we now face is from the cumulative buildup of these toxins in our bodies and the harmful effects these chemicals have on our health. And it's not just a "little" toxicity, either. Today humans roam the earth with an average of 700 or more industrial chemicals flowing through their bodies. That's an estimate, of course, because no one really knows for sure. (For most chemicals in circulation today, no technology even exists yet to detect their presence in the human body.) The vast major-ity of these chemicals, which are commonplace today, hadn't even been created in a laboratory until 40 to 50 years ago.

There are also countless, naturally occurring toxins in our envi-ronment. On any given day, we can be exposed to organic bio-toxins or inorganic toxins, such as poisonous chemicals and other danger-ous man-made substances. Ultimately, all toxins can take a serious toll on our health. Some display cancer-causing properties that could potentially kill us.

Damage can result quickly from exposure to a large or highly concentrated dangerous pollutant. Frequently and more insidiously, damage results from a gradual accumulation of smaller amounts of less-potent toxins from a variety of sources. This is often referred to as "chronic toxic overload," or "the body's toxic burden," or simply "the body burden."

There are multiple definitions of toxins and toxicity, as well as for a number of sub-categories. Let's start with the definition for "toxicity." It is the degree to which a substance (a toxin or a poison) can harm humans or animals. The various levels of toxicity include:

- **Acute toxicity**—refers to the harmful effects in an organism through single or short-term exposure.

- **Sub-chronic toxicity**—defined as the ability of a toxic substance to cause effects for more than one year but less than the lifetime of the exposed organism.

- **Chronic toxicity**—the ability of a substance or mixture of substances to cause harmful effects over an extended period, usually upon repeated or continuous exposure. Sometimes chronic toxicity will last the entire life of the exposed organism.

Toxins are identified as chemical, biological, bacterial, physical, or caused by radiation. These are some of the more prevalent ones:

- **Chemical toxicants**—inorganic substances such as lead, mercury, asbestos, hydrofluoric acid, chlorine gas, and organic compounds such as methyl alcohol, most medications, and poisons from living things.

- **Biological toxicants**—bacteria and viruses that can induce disease in living organisms. Biological toxicity is tricky to measure because the "threshold dose" may be a single organism. One virus, bacterium, or worm can, theoretically, reproduce to cause serious infection.

- **Physical toxicants**—substances that can interfere with the body's natural processes because of their physical nature. For example, coal dust and asbestos can be fatal if they are inhaled.

- **Radiation**—can have a toxic effect on organisms.

FOUR WAYS THAT TOXINS ENTER YOUR BODY

We absorb toxins in four primary ways: through the air we breathe, the water we drink and bathe in, the food we eat, and the many personal care or beauty products we apply. It's basically impossible to completely avoid them. We are surrounded by polluted air and contaminated water, and our food is full of pesticides, chemicals, and additives. And even if we swear off cosmetics, most of us still use the bare essentials like soap, deodorant, and toothpaste, all of which contain harmful substances.

Breathing Air

The first portal through which the body receives toxins is in the air we breathe. Thanks to the waste that we produce and the chemical by-products of our modern lifestyle, this planet continues to become more and more hostile to all life forms—especially us.

We dump thousands of tons of pollution into the sky and ground 365 days a year. Coal-fired power plants not only supply our power grid with electricity but are also the biggest source of harmful air pollution compared to all other sources of industrial pollution. In fact, the American Lung Association estimates that more than 386,000 tons of 84 different pollutants are emitted into the air from more than 400 different power plants in 46 states.[18]

You are not safe from polluted air whether you are in your home or vacationing in the Arctic Circle. The air supply on this planet is under attack by pollution created from our gigantic manufacturing facilities and the cars we drive. Even secondhand cigarette smoke can be a challenge to avoid, whether you smoke or not.

Not all has to be doom and gloom. You will learn in our second book, *TDOS Solutions*, the ways to deal with the accumulation of airborne toxins to more manageable levels.

We've seen stories appearing from Beijing showing thousands of people early in the morning in front of these huge TV screens. The people were wearing masks and watching a virtual sunrise on the TV screens, as the air pollution was so severe it had blocked out the sun. Is this air pollution coming to a city near you? Maybe not, but the pollution from China is being carried by airborne currents across the Pacific Ocean and contribute to pollution in the Western United States.

Absorbing Water

The second major source of toxic infiltration is our water supply. Whether we're drinking water or bathing in it, we are drowning ourselves in this toxic soup. Tap water is teeming with toxins!

The Environmental Working Group conducted a study and discovered that on any given day there are more than 140 contaminants in common household tap water. In addition, over the past few years, studies have revealed that a number of pharmaceuticals—both over-the-counter and prescription drugs—are appearing in our water tables. Some of the most common drugs found in water include antibiotics, anti-depressants, birth control pills, seizure medications, cancer treatments, prescription painkillers, tranquilizers, and cholesterol-lowering compounds.

So here is something you were probably not expecting to read: Don't drink tap water. If possible, avoid most sources of tap water: at home, in the office, in city parks and theme parks, and in restaurants. The bottom line is that our water sources are loaded with chemicals and should be avoided at all costs.

Tests have been developed to detect more than 315 pollutants in the tap water accessible to the American population. This was based on a study conducted by the Environmental Working Group (EWG) and their analysis of almost 20 million records obtained from state water officials. The reason for this contamination is that municipal water treatment plants are not technologically advanced enough to remove all of the toxins.

We know it sounds daunting, but the good news is that we *can* fight back. After all, one of the few things we still have control over in our lives is what we choose to put into our bodies. If you must use tap water, get a water purifier with a simple filter. Fortunately, accessing clean water can be done fairly easily and is more cost effective than ever thanks to more and more people leading the charge away from drinking unfiltered tap water. (Read more on these and other solutions in our next book.)

Eating Food

So the air is polluted and the water is poisoned, but how does our food supply hold up in this equation? Sadly, food is perhaps the biggest culprit in the toxic arena. Our food supply has more toxins than you may realize. Even organic foods can't escape high levels of pesticides, chemicals, and other pollutants. One of the major offenders for toxic exposure is processed foods. These foods are full of chemicals and additives that can create symptoms ranging from increased hunger cravings and weight gain to poor digestive health and allergies.

There are thousands of chemicals used in the production of our foods each day, according to the book *The Hundred Year Lie: How to Protect Yourself from the Chemicals that Are Killing You* by Randall Fitzgerald. Most have never been tested for how they might harm us. The food industry utilizes artificial colorings, fillers, additives, and untold numbers of chemicals to improve everything from the look, taste, and consistency of our foods. It's done to create a tastier, more appealing "product," but it's also done to increase sales with almost zero regard to the possible health consequences.

Let's remember that the financial bottom line is what really matters most to the food industry. If we come back for a second or third helping—enticed by the way these "foods" have been chemically altered, tweaked, and engineered—then these food chemists have won. Essentially, they increase profit margins with no regard to the havoc that "special ingredients" may have on our health—as individuals, as a nation, and as a species.

If you want to limit the amount of toxins you are ingesting through food, consume a whole foods diet with plenty of organic meats and vegetables. Avoid processed foods at all costs, and pay careful attention to food labels and ingredient lists.

Applying Beauty and Healthcare Products

Beauty and personal care products we choose to put "on" us can be as toxic as the foods we put "in" us. Everyday products we use to look our best may actually be the greatest source of aging and health challenges. That's because most deodorants, toothpastes, lotions, soaps, hair products, fragrances, and cosmetics are full of toxic chemicals.

The personal care and cosmetic products we use every day have more than 10,000 chemicals included in their ingredient lists that have not been tested by the Food and Drug Administration (FDA). Few of these have been tested for the harm they might cause us. The FDA treats these manufacturers as if they are on the honor system. If the companies say the products are safe, the FDA gives their approval. It all comes back full circle to profit. Imagine the cost of testing all these chemicals—the time involved, the sales, and profits—all lost. Let's face it; safety just isn't a lucrative business!

If you really want to know how toxic your cosmetics are, visit this great website www.ewg.org and search beauty secrets. This site will reveal to you, by brand name and type, how toxic the cosmetics you apply really are. Search for alternative options that are less harmful.

FIRST STUDIES ON HUMANS AND TOXINS

Aside from the blood testing performed in 2000 by the Centers for Disease Control and Prevention, the Mount Sinai Medical School in New York was the first nongovernment entity to initiate tests for toxins using human test subjects in 2005. The results found that the test subjects had, at a minimum, an average of 91 toxic compound traces in their blood and urine. These included:

- 76 chemicals linked to cancer causation
- 77 that are toxic to the immune system
- 79 associated with birth defects
- 77 toxic chemicals that are potentially detrimental to the reproductive system

Unborn children are not even safe from all the toxins in our environment, despite what scientists once thought. It was common belief that the placenta kept babies safe from most environmental pollutants and chemicals, but the Environmental Working Group conducted an investigation and discovered that this isn't the case. Researchers from two labs tested umbilical cord blood from ten babies born in hospitals in the US in August and September 2004. They found pesticides, coal waste, and ingredients from consumer products, gasoline, and even garbage in the cord blood. The study revealed that newborns enter the world with an average of 200 chemicals in their tiny bodies, which may be a conservative estimate.[19]

Included in the toxins researchers were able to identify were eight different chemicals used in packaging for fast food, clothing, and textiles; the chemical marketed by DuPont as Teflon, which is believed to be a human carcinogen, according to the EPA's Science Advisory Board; dozens of flame retardants and their byproducts; and a broad range of pesticides. Of the 287 chemicals researchers discovered in umbilical cord blood, 180 are known to cause cancer, 217 cause brain and nervous system toxicity, and 208 cause birth defects or abnormal development. What these chemicals do synergistically, when mixed together, remains mostly unexplored territory, though as you will see below, a body of alarming research data is emerging.

In addition to all the vital nutrients a developing baby needs, the umbilical cord is also carrying a flood of toxins across the placenta. This can't be good for the future of human health and the survival of our species.[20]

Unfortunately, we have only ourselves to blame. Mankind has created this toxic world we live in. Moreover, what's significant is that we should have seen the warning signs that were "posted" in the form of our failing health and declining air quality; the fact is that a lot of this has been done and occurred without our permission or consent.

TOXIN MIXTURES AND THEIR SYNERGIES UNDERMINE HEALTH

Here is a representative sampling of the research data accumulating over the past decade, revealing some of the dangers and health impacts from toxic synergies that many of us are being exposed to on a daily basis.

Even low-dose, "non-toxic" chemical synergies can trigger cancer. The International Agency for Research on Cancer estimates that up to 19 percent of all human cancers are caused by exposures to toxins in the environment. That percentage estimate should increase significantly given the following findings that illustrate how low-dose levels of certain chemicals, which may be harmless by themselves, become cancer-causing when mixed together. To determine which low-dose exposures to certain ordinarily non-toxic chemicals might cause cancer, 85 chemicals were reviewed by a team of scientists for the cancer medical journal *Carcinogenesis*. Nearly 60 percent of these chemicals exerted low-dose effects. The scientists concluded: "Our analysis suggests that the cumulative effects of individual (noncarcinogenic) chemicals acting on different pathways, and a variety of related systems, organs, tissues and cells, could plausibly conspire to produce carcinogenic synergies."[21]

Two contaminants interact synergistically in ground water. Contamination of ground water with arsenic is widespread, and now, with ever greater use of dichlorvos—an organophosphate insecticide applied in agriculture—these two contaminants are mixing together and posing a danger to people who come in contact with the irrigation water or who eat the non-organic crops grown in contaminated water. To assess the "synergistic interactions" or "joint toxic" actions among these toxicants," researchers reviewed the science literature on exposure and found "serious concerns" about the bioavailability (human tissue absorption) of the contaminants and a possible long list of health problems the two could cause by acting synergistically. "Dreadfully very few studies are available on combined exposures to these toxicants on the animal or human system," warned the scientists.[22]

Insecticides and herbicides combine to produce toxic synergies. Chinese scientists examined different combinations of five common insecticides, two common herbicides, and the heavy metal cadmium found in soil to determine how toxic these combinations are to life forms. They found "synergistic effects predominated at lower effect levels; the patterns of interactions found in six, seven, and eight-component mixture displayed synergism." In other words, the more chemicals that interacted, the greater the toxicity produced in the environment.[23]

Even sunlight can transform harmless into harmful. When sunlight or electromagnetic fields interact with chemicals, such as pesticides, synergistic mixture effects can occur. "The cocktail of sunlight irradiated sulcotrione pesticide has a greater {toxicity} than the parent molecule," wrote one science team, citing but one of many examples. They urge that "synergy in living organisms" be made a priority for study, starting with evaluations of the multiple environmental contamination issues raised by chemical cocktails, and radiation exposure.[24]

Low dose chemical synergies need to be studied. In a review of the study literature on chemical mixtures and synergies, 90 studies were identified by one research team, writing in the journal

Critical Reviews Toxicology. They reported that "few included quantitative estimates of low-dose synergy." The vast majority of the studies evaluated high doses of chemicals interacting, when those are only the "tip of the iceberg" when it comes to what is possibly going on with the low-dose mixtures.[25]

Neurobehavioral problems can occur from common chemical interactions. Animal studies with applications to humans found that certain chemicals can interact to create synergies that affect neonatal brain development, resulting in behavioral disorders. In a study from the journal *Toxicological Science*, it was found that PBDEs, a chemical used as flame-retardants in many textiles, can interact with PCBs and DDT, in the environment from industrial processes, to trigger and enhance brain developmental problems for humans.[26]

Food additives synergize to cause ADHD. In testing the combined toxicity of various food additives, commonly found in processed foods for children, a team of British scientists found "significant synergy observed between combinations of Brilliant Blue (a food coloring) with L-glutamic acid, and Quinoline Yellow with aspartame (a food flavoring.)" These additives, typically found in snacks and drinks, together create cellular toxicity sufficient to stunt nerve cell growth.[27]

Combined pollutants intensify diabetes risk. Each of six persistent organic pollutants—PCBs, two types of dioxins, two pesticides, and DDE—can on their own, given the dose exposure, cause type 2 diabetes in humans. When exposure occurs to these pollutants in combination, the risk for diabetes skyrockets. In 2,016 people tested, 80 percent of them had detectable amounts of these contaminants. People with the highest levels of these contaminants were 38 times more likely to contract diabetes. This chemical synergy inside people's bodies may be one reason why the number of Americans with diabetes more than doubled between 1980 and 2004.[28]

SUPERBUGS AND ANTIBIOTICS

How aware are you of the amount of antibiotics you consume in your diet—antibiotics that are not prescribed by your doctor? You absorb them simply by eating food comprised of animals that have been injected with antibiotics.

In his book *The Omnivore's Dilemma*, Michael Pollan pointed out that whatever a plant or animal eats, we eat, when we consume the plant or animal. This, of course includes antibiotics, animal growth hormones, herbicides, pesticides, and GMOs (genetically modified organisms).

With everything out there invading our bodies, our miraculous immune systems have gone to extreme measures to combat viruses, bacteria, and other invaders. As our bodies evolve to combat these organisms, these little monsters are evolving as well. Who will eventually win this battle? Who will prevail in Mother Nature's survival of the fittest?

Consider how the body's already-maxed-out immune system is working overtime to combat these toxic burdens, including superbugs. "Health officials are raising concerns that it may soon be too late to stop superbugs," warned a *USA Today* article in 2013. The story describes a "superbug" as a resistant organism that is untreatable and potentially deadly. The "superbugs" are spreading through the worst possible places—hospitals and nursing homes. The places we go to get well may just be making us sicker than ever.

Not only are these superbugs resistant to antibiotics but they are also capable of spreading their resistance to other bacteria. With this potentially lethal combination, superbugs prey on the most vulnerable: people with pre-existing infections and weakened immune systems. When these mini monsters enter this at-risk population, only about half of these patients survive. The repercussions of something so deadly that also has the capacity to transfer its lethal characteristics to other bacteria could potentially mean devastating results for the general population. Even common infections could become untreatable.

Again, what if what we think is working . . . isn't? In fact, what if it's making things worse? Consider this: With only 10 percent of the world's population, North America consumes 50 percent of the world's antibiotics. This overuse of antibiotics is only partially because of over prescribing. Roughly 80 percent of these antibiotics are used in feed for the animals that make up our food supply.[29]

"You are what you eat," has never been truer than in this day and age of modified, enhanced, and contaminated foodstuffs. Think about what you ate for breakfast or lunch today. Can you even pronounce the ingredients listed on the packaging? Do we know exactly what was fed to that rib eye sitting on our dinner plate? Now, more than ever, it's important to purchase organic meats that are free of hormones and antibiotics.

So who is going to win this battle, the bugs or the humans? Can we depend on the scientists to remain one step ahead of these invasive organisms? The same formulas of antibiotics that have been effective for so long are now exposing their weaknesses.

The combination of antibiotic-resistant superbugs and toxins loaded in our bodies from what we inhale, drink, and eat, food lacking in nutrition, and stress, stress, stress all create a perfect storm for our health. But no one is telling you how all these factors interconnect and magnify to the detriment of your health. At least, no one was . . . until now.

YOUR BODY CAN ONLY TAKE SO MUCH ABUSE

The human body is a masterpiece of engineering. It has been constructed to detoxify itself of impurities with help from the liver, lungs, kidneys, and lymphatic system all working in collaboration. However, just like when design specifications are exceeded in human-engineered machines, breakdown occurs when there is an "overload" on the system. In the case of the human body, "breakdown" is manifested in inadequate organ function and chronic disease. Toxins are playing a major role in the collapse of the body's functions. Until we reduce their numbers, the symptoms will continue. Disease numbers are on the rise. Although we are living longer, we are living sicker.

Western medicine has made tremendous strides in prolonging life with advancements in surgical technologies and medications. While this may have added to the "quantity" of our lives (i.e., living longer), this has occurred at the expense of our "quality" of life. This does not seem like a smart trade-off. It makes no sense to extend your life if you lose the quality to enjoy the things that make life worth living. There must be a connection between toxins and the changes in the population's "healthy living."

You can question the correlation between toxic exposure and the effects on human health but the evidence is worth reviewing carefully. There are new research studies on the long-term health effects of what has previously been deemed as "relatively harmless." Toxins are more than just a little worrisome. Scientists are discovering that continued exposure to common, non-lethal toxins can negatively affect major body systems. Britain's Environmental Toxins Foundation has stated that there is "mounting evidence of structural and genetic damage, potentially caused to the human morphology, through the huge influx of chemical agents found in the air, soil and water today."

What kind of cumulative damage? One widely acknowledged example would be high cholesterol and triglyceride levels which are, in and of themselves, non-lethal. However, over time, together they can be a causative factor in a lethal heart attack.

It is time to apply the same thought process to toxins and toxicants.

AN OVERWHELMED DEFENSE SYSTEM

The human body has had to adapt over generations to remove various toxic loads. As mentioned earlier, the body is equipped with powerful detoxification and cleansing systems in the liver, stomach, intestines, and kidneys as a means of protecting itself. The liver is our primary detoxification organ, metabolizing thousands of different chemicals that humans are exposed to daily. Much of what is eaten must pass through the liver. As the liver breaks down nutrients, it also metabolizes toxic substances. In most cases, these toxins are cleared from the blood and eliminated in bile or urine, but in other cases they can be stored in fat.

The body stores these impurities in body tissues such as fat even as polluted elements continue to enter the body. The fat cells then enlarge because of additional fat, and the toxins are "solubilized" with the fat. According to Dr. Mark Hyman, there are two types of toxins when it comes to storage in the body: water soluble or fat-soluble. Water-soluble toxins will be eliminated through urine and sweat. Fat-soluble toxins will dissolve and recombine using fat.

After extensive research in recent years, scientists have begun to realize that the long-term implications of toxins may result in drastic changes to the internal structure of the human body. The immune system is incapable of dealing with so many chemicals, and the latest evidence reveals that toxins disrupt metabolism. When the body does not metabolize effectively, this can lead to overweight and obesity. The American Society of Endocrinologists coined a new term for these chemicals: obesogens. These obesogens are foreign chemical compounds that disrupt normal development and balance of fat metabolism.

The Endocrine Society, the largest organization of experts devoted to research on hormones and the clinical practice of endocrinology, reports that "the rise in the incidence in obesity matches the rise in the use and distribution of industrial chemicals that may be playing a role in a generation of obesity, suggesting Endocrine Disrupting Chemicals (EDCs) may be linked to this epidemic." Endocrine disrupting chemicals (EDCs) are a type of obesogen, a term broadly defined as chemicals that can interfere with hormone action. These EDCs play havoc in our bodies in many ways. For example, it is now clear that other hormone receptor types and functions, including those involved in metabolism, obesity, and brain signaling can be targets of EDCs.

According to 2009 and 2010 reports from the Endocrine Society, increasing levels of obesity may be linked with the increase in use of industrial chemicals. Researchers with the organization believe EDCs could be responsible. They enter our bodies from numerous sources, including so-called "natural" compounds like those in soy products, food packaging, processed foods, and the pesticides that are sprayed on our fruit and vegetables. It's believed that these chemicals take over the natural bodily systems that control our body weight, actually causing us to gain weight.

HOW TOXINS TRIGGER WEIGHT PROBLEMS

Chemicals and toxins are stored in the body's fat cells. The fat we really need to fear is the visceral fat that collects around the organs in the abdomen. Visceral fat produces pro-inflammatory mediators, which have been linked to cardiovascular disease, diabetes, and certain cancers. The journal of Hepatology (11 April 2008) reports evidence that visceral fat is linked to nonalcoholic fatty liver disease and metabolic syndrome. This visceral fat therefore causes stress in the body, resulting in a release of the hormone cortisol. Cortisol's job is to manage stress in the body. With every give, there must be a take. The main side effect of cortisol is that when its levels are raised in the body, the body shuts off its natural method of burning fat. This prevents weight loss.

The United States is beginning to see the repercussions of wading in this toxic soup. There is no doubt that the waistline in this country has expanded. The numbers of overweight and obese people have reached epidemic levels. It is clear that the interconnectivity between toxicity, nutritional deficiency, and stress are all contributing co-factors to this worldwide problem. Nutritional deficiency allows toxins to accumulate in the body. Without proper nutrients, the body's natural defenses and ability to rid itself of this toxic fat is greatly diminished.

We know that obesogens, caused by toxicity and nutritional deficiency, are helping notch a new hole in an old belt in the human body. These obesogens are promoting weight gain in the body as a defense system. The body is smart and realizes there are foreign substances battling to do as much damage as possible. A lack of proper nutrition gives the body no resources to eliminate these toxins naturally. So the human body builds fat cells to protect itself from the chemicals. Obesogens are programming us to be overweight, as you will learn in chapter three of this book.

TOXINS COULD BECOME THE TOP KILLER OF THE 21ST CENTURY

In our view, toxins will prove to be *the* big killers in the twenty-first century. And we're not alone. According to Dr. Rick Irvin, a toxicologist at Texas A&M University, "Chemicals have replaced bacteria and viruses as the main threat to human health. The diseases we are beginning to see as the major cause of death in the latter part of the twentieth century and into the twenty-first century are diseases of chemical origins." We are now potentially faced with a major toxic impact, and a lack of awareness or intervention from either federal or local authorities. Combine this level of toxicity with the nutritional deficiency crisis (identified in the next chapter), and the toxins are running out of control without nutrition to lighten the toxic load.

The toxins are running rampant while the body's available intervention-nutrition designed to clear the toxins is absent. In our current nutritionally deficient state, the body cannot rid itself of the toxins. The body needs a massive amount of nutrients in today's world for us to have even a fighting chance against this toxic army that is overwhelming our nearly defenseless bodies.

Why does the body have such a problem fighting these toxins? It has become clear that with our nutritionally bankrupt food supply, we lack sufficient nutrition—actual, healthy, natural, non-toxic nutrients. Without these nutrients, the body does not have the fuel it so desperately needs to combat this onslaught of toxicity. We're not hungry—far from it. What we are is "overfed and undernourished," which means our bellies might be full and our waistlines expanding, but our bodies are hungry for more and better, *healthier* nutrients.

We now have fewer antioxidants in our food supply, which are vital weapons in the fight against the free radicals that are being created by toxins. Why does this matter? These free radicals lead to oxidative stress, which greatly accelerates the process of decay of the body's cells. Simply put, when the body's toxic load becomes greater than its ability to adapt to it, let alone fight it, the body's overall health will suffer the consequences.

The body creates its own version of what we call toxin "hunters." These are naturally occurring nutrients that assist the body in breaking down toxins into soluble substances so the body can safely pass them out through the liver, kidneys, and finally through the colon. However, the body can't produce sufficient quantities of these natural toxin hunters due to our nutritional deficiency (insufficiency).

The fact that toxins can be dangerous to our health has been known for quite some time. However, our understanding of how even low-level toxic exposure threatens our health and to what extent is only now being examined. Evidence is at last building about the effects of our toxic environment on our long-term health and toxins' role in chronic diseases. Although scientists have known for quite a while that pollution and pesticides can adversely affect human health, mounting evidence reveals far more deadly connections between toxic exposure and a variety of diseases than was previously expected.

The most disturbing discovery is that chronic exposure to even low levels of common toxins can have long-term negative health effects. This is because, despite their low level, toxins accumulate in our bodies over time, damaging the neurological, immune, and endocrine systems in the process.

To complicate matters further, many governments and health organizations do not seem to be addressing this serious problem sufficiently, if at all. Without accountability and cleanup programs, the toxic exposure overload continues to spiral out of control.

The harmful effects of low levels of contaminants can usually be determined after many years of analysis. Sometimes occupational diseases provide clues about environmental contaminants. The Romans were aware that lead could cause serious health problems, like mental illness and even death, so they used slaves to mine the lead for their pipes. The expression "mad as a hatter" originated from the neurological damage and mental confusion suffered by workers who cured felt with mercury compounds in the manufacturing of hats. In modern times, it has been recognized that inhaling asbestos, coal dust, cotton fiber dust, and tobacco smoke can result in decreased lung function, cancer, and death.

The danger of toxins lies in the fact that they are invisible, so they are not easily avoided. Likewise, their effects do not surface immediately, so the damage does not necessarily deter repeat exposure. You feel okay, so what's the big problem? Just because a toxin won't cause immediate death or severe organ shutdown doesn't mean it is not dangerous, or that the body is any better equipped to deal with it.

The research doesn't lie. There are sobering new discoveries being made every day regarding the studies linking deterioration of our health to toxins. The results of these studies are more than a little unsettling. Lead exposure, alone, has been linked to cancer, cardiovascular disease, stroke, heart attacks, renal failure, osteoporosis, and macular degeneration.

"IT COULDN'T HAPPEN TO ME!"

You may be thinking, "I live in a safe, clean environment, don't I? None of this could ever happen to me, could it?" It no longer matters where you live. You may be exposed to harmful substances every day because many of these chemicals are used in farming, food production, and consumer goods manufacturing. You may not work in a mine or live next to a nuclear plant but the food that gets shipped, handled, or served to you every day is full of toxins you cannot see and certainly cannot taste.

Toxins migrate. Their molecules hitchhike on the wind, attached to dust particles. Once released into the environment, they can travel through the water. For example, polychlorinated biphenyls (PCBs) and polybrominated diphenyl ethers (PBDEs), which are used widely as flame-retardant additives in polyurethane foam for carpet padding, mattresses, chairs, sofas, and other furniture, have been found in the food supply, including fish and many animal fats. These fire retardants have also been detected in humans and in human breast milk across the planet. These are endocrine-disrupting compounds with the potential to profoundly affect sexual development. So the result of this migration is that no one on the planet can be considered immune to contact with toxins, or the absorption of toxins, whether you live in the cold Arctic or the hot Sahara Desert.

There is no escape from the toxic onslaught we are faced with in this world. There is no quiet corner of the earth that has yet to be taken over by this toxic burden. We know that toxic molecules are in our favorite destination regions and even the world's most remote areas. No one is immune to the threat.

HEALTH CARE IN CRISIS

As our population gets sicker at younger and younger ages, the medical community seems ill-prepared to manage the health-care crisis that looms as a result. Imagine in the future, legions of the sick marching on the hospitals when there may not be enough money, beds, drugs, or doctors. Don't depend solely on the current medical establishment for the only solution.

New health care legislation is giving 30 million more people access to health care in this country. Yet this new development comes just as we are facing a dwindling number of doctors. The Association of American Medical Colleges' (AAMC) Center for Workforce Studies estimated that we will be 130,000 physicians short for the needs of our country by the year 2025. It is time for everyone to become aware, get involved, and make their decisions.

What about the use of herbicides, pesticides, and GMOs? Future historians will look back and write about our time, not about how many pounds of pesticides we did or did not apply but about how willing we are to sacrifice our children and jeopardize future generations with this massive experiment that is based on false promises and flawed science just to benefit the bottom line of a commercial enterprise.

Dr. Don Huber, Professor Emeritus at Purdue University, is a featured lecturer on the impact of the herbacide glyphosate used on our crops and its connection to the health of livestock and humans. As one of the world's leading authorities on soil, he talks and writes about the devastating effects of these chemicals and the ingestion of foods with Genetically Modified Organisms (GMOs). This use of this in our agriculture is a frightening worldwide experiment. We are seeing signs that our government should never have allowed this situation to start in the first place. We may eventually come to realize that we have already sealed the fate of future generations.

There is no doubt we are playing a deadly game of roulette with our future. We are realizing that the womb is no longer safe from the outside world. Pesticides created with the intent to maximize profits are now posing a risk to the future of the world.

One of the best sources for information on GMO's effects is Jeffrey Smith, a leading researcher on GMOs in the world. His book and documentary *Genetic Roulette* is truly eye opening. For up-to-date information on GMO Research at his Institute for Responsible Technology visit www.responsibletechnology.org.

Some of the chemicals that are all around us have the ability to interfere with our endocrine systems, which regulate the hormones that control our weight, biorhythms, and reproduction. Lab studies have shown that low levels of endocrine-disrupting chemicals induce subtle changes in the developing fetus that have profound health effects in adulthood and even on subsequent generations.

The chemicals ingested daily by a pregnant woman may affect her unborn child, since fetuses and newborns lack the functional enzymes in the liver and other organs to break down such chemicals. In the past several decades, animal studies have shown that these chemicals can disrupt hormones and brain development.

These toxins and chemicals are truly widespread. There is no question that the damage we are doing to our bodies—and our communities—is much bigger than on the individual level and is indeed on a global scale. This is a problem that our families will encounter for years to come.

> "We don't know the future effects of these toxins on generations to come. It is too early in the game to see the large amount of damage being inflicted on new lives. The argument that toxins would be destroyed in the gut is far from true. All you have to do is look at what is being passed into the bloodstream. We may be doing irreparable harm to our future children."
>
> **—JEFFREY SMITH**
> *Genetic Roulette: The Documented Health Risks of Genetically Engineered Food*

This toxic crisis may already be emerging with significant impacts in our youth. According to the American Diabetes Association, one in every three babies born in the United States today will now develop diabetes within their lifetimes. That's 33 percent of humans born in the United States! A single statistic like that could undermine our health care system. We have also seen a rise in autism of roughly 3,000 percent since 1990 as well as rising levels of sexual development in prepubescent girls. These are shocking statistics for the new millennium.

With this toxic "gift that keeps on giving," we owe it to ourselves to be informed about what these toxins are doing to us. We owe it to new mothers everywhere, who want to give their babies the best possible chance of growing into healthy adults; we owe it to our children, the next generation.

AWARENESS IS CRITICAL

There is a problem: Who is out there to protect us? The first answer should be you. It is up to each one of us to stay informed and make the best decisions for our own health, along with the health of our families. But we can't do it alone. The US Food and Drug Administration and the US Environmental Protection Agency are federal agencies established to protect us. Together they are responsible for banning dangerous chemicals and making sure our food and drugs have been thoroughly tested. Scientists and clinicians across diverse disciplines are concerned that the efforts of the FDA and EPA are insufficient in terms of the complex cocktail of chemicals present in our daily lives. At a minimum, more suitable screening and testing is needed with regard to endocrine disrupting chemicals. The need for such tests has been recognized for more than a decade but there is still no sound testing protocol. One word for this shocking lack of a sound protocol is *scary*. If we do nothing to avoid these toxins, then we should not be surprised at the possible outcome.

Toxicity, nutritional deficiency, being overweight, and stress are all realities in our world today. Each is significant in and of itself, but they are interrelated and exacerbate one another in ways that we are only now just beginning to understand.

The four TDOS co-factors affect one another, magnifying their negative impacts and ultimately our health and wellness potential. There is little doubt that we are now living in toxic bodies. The potential problems caused by toxicity, this first co-factor, are for the first time being studied.

Our current health-care delivery system is defensive in its nature. There has to be a new solution. Hopefully, some of the evidence presented so far has opened your eyes to looking at your health management as an offensive strategy. Specifically, we need new nutritional approaches that are equipped to fight toxicity in the body. So much has changed in the last 30 years alone. It is almost impossible to compare now and then based on nutrition.

We live in a world processed for speed. Everything has been made for our convenience, especially our meals. It's time to step back and examine how those meals were prepared and, in some cases, go even further and look at details like the food packaging itself. There is no doubt that the environment we live in right now is toxic and it is our responsibility to find the solutions.

The evidence proves toxicity's role as a major contributing co-factor to being or becoming overweight. Once the body is overweight, that becomes a contributing co-factor to stress in the body. The heart and other organs have to work harder to carry out their functions. The more overweight you are, the more difficult the job becomes.

When adding all of this together, the TDOS Syndrome makes it harder to maintain and increase your overall health and maximize your wellness potential. A healthier lifestyle always begins with awareness, and being open to the possibility that what you think you know may not be true, as this book will endeavor to show you.

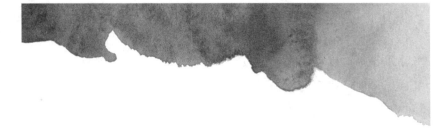

PART TWO

Co-Factor D—
The Deficiency
of Nutrients

Co-Factor D—
The Deficiency of Nutrients

*A Serious Depletion with Serious Effects on
Our Potential to Have a High Quality of Life*

Life has blessed me with two wonderful sons: Drew, a coauthor on all of my books, and Colin, an articulate spokesperson for my research. Colin was a gifted 20-year-old athlete who seemed to have everything going for him. Unfortunately, he had an inability to concentrate, as do many young people today. He was on powerful drugs to deal with his condition that, at times, was so severe that he would say he had nothing to live for. Colin could not tolerate being on his medication, and so he felt trapped by his situation. As a father, I was heartbroken and terrified.

Fortunately, in 2003, after I had my own miraculous health turn around, I met Dr. John Gray, author of *Men Are from Mars and Women Are from Venus*. John had also lost close to 30 pounds utilizing the same nutritional approach I had used. As we talked, I shared Colin's struggles with him. John recommended that I put Colin on our nutritional regimen. I explained that Colin didn't need to lose weight; he was an all-state basketball player and in excellent shape. John reminded me that weight loss was a side benefit to the central reason for the natural detox protocol—restoring the body's nutritional balance and health.

Colin started on the protocol reluctantly. In less than a week, however, Colin told me, with tears in his eyes, "Dad, I don't know what's in this stuff but I feel better than I have since I was a little kid. This may really be an answer to my struggles."

It turned out that Colin had a deficiency in copper, zinc, and lithium orotate, due to his nutritionally deficient eating habits. By correcting that with supplementation, he was able to counteract the deficiency and regain his ability to focus with clarity. John Gray has become a mentor and friend and now, a decade later, he has shared Colin's story with hundreds of other parents, helping many kids to recover from a similar attention deficit disorder condition.

Colin and I both had do-overs. We were able to hit the reset button, thanks to our discovery that we were starved for nutrients that were lacking in our diets. We all suffer from a nutrient depletion not only because we are often consuming processed foods void of any vitamins and minerals, but also because our very soil has been stripped of essential nutrients. It's important that we consume plenty of trace elements, vitamins, minerals, and high quality protein to support our body's detoxification mechanism.

OUR FOOD SUPPLY HAS BEEN "DUMBED DOWN"

Nutritional deficiency (or insufficiency) competes with toxins as the stealthiest individual factor of the health-undermining TDOS Syndrome. It's stealthy because, like toxins, nutrients must be measured, since they aren't visible to the naked eye, and these measurements must be interpreted properly by medical specialists to signal the depth and gravity of any threat to health. The physical effects of too many toxins and too few essential nutrients surface over time as the manifestations of illness and disease. But too few mainstream medical professionals are trained to recognize the interconnections.

Nutrients constitute the "intelligence" animating our food supply, acting to reinforce human health and providing preventive medicine. As Hippocrates, the ancient Greek "father of medicine," advised: "Let thy food by thy medicine." Without adequate nutrition, the existence of the human race would become a side note in the planet's history. A high level of nutritional deficiency may open the door to usher in other health problems for humanity that we haven't even detected yet, particularly because so many people have become more concerned about convenience than health when making food choices.

The "dumbing down" of our food supply began in earnest with the wholesale introduction of agricultural techniques in the 20th century that relied on chemical engineering to increase harvests. This "dumbing" was accelerated and intensified by the widespread processing of crops and animals into convenience foods and fast-food categories of edible products.

THE THREE STEPS OF NUTRITIONAL DEPLETION

We can divide the nutrient loss in our food supply into three steps of depletion: loss from agricultural practices, loss through processing, and loss through cooking. Aggressive farming practices and the increasing use of pesticides has reduced the quality of our soil so that it contains fewer minerals, which means that the fruits and vegetables grown in that soil have become more nutrient deficient. We then lose even more nutrients during food processing and certain cooking techniques.

Nutrient Loss from Agricultural Practices

What may have been the first public alert about soil depletion, and the resulting loss of nutrients in crops, emerged in a 1936 report published by a committee of the US Senate. The report, based on research by soil scientist Dr. Charles Northen, raised this provocative question: "Do you know that most of us today are suffering from certain dangerous diet deficiencies which cannot be remedied until the depleted soils from which our foods come are brought into proper mineral balance?" By pointing out the dietary deficiencies that result from the nutrient depletion occurring in our crop soils, this government state-ment proved predictive and prophetic. It was a warning mostly ignored for a half-century.

After many years of aggressive farming, use of pesticides, and stripping off topsoil, we depleted the essential nutrients in our crops. If our food supply was labeled nearly bankrupt of essential minerals 75 years ago, there is a strong chance we have a far worse situation today.

To underscore the severity of the problem, a United Nations Con-ference on Environment and Development issued an Earth Summit Report in 1992 that raised this alarm: "there is deep concern over continuing major declines in the mineral values in farm and range soils throughout the world." The primary soil depletion culprit was identified at that time as the application of artificial chemical fertil-izers, though other studies have since revealed that added mineral depletion occurs as a result of acid rain, caused by air pollutants, which particularly affect calcium and magnesium levels in the soil.[30] Plants that used to absorb 70 to 80 different minerals from the soil dramati-cally reduced the numbers and amounts of the minerals absorbed after contact with these chemicals, which greatly increased crop yields at the expense of soil degradation.

The 1992 Earth Summit Report provided the following estimated soil mineral depletion levels (percentages) over the past 100 years:[31]

North America	85%
South America	76%
Europe	72%
Asia	76%
Africa	74%
Australia	55%

Food scientists compared the mineral content of 20 fruits and 20 vegetables grown in the 1930s on through the 1980s and discovered numerous substantial reductions in mineral content. There were significant reductions, for instance, in the levels of calcium, magnesium, copper, and sodium in vegetables and magnesium, iron, copper, and potassium in fruit. The only mineral over the 50-year period that showed no significant difference or decline was phosphorus. The food scientists, writing in the *British Food Journal*, expressed the belief that these nutrient declines were probably caused by changes in agricultural practices.[32]

Research published in the *Journal of the American College of Nutrition* in 2004 further revealed how widespread vitamin and mineral deficiencies have become in our food supply. This study found serious decreases in the mineral and vitamin content of 43 garden crops grown in US markets during the period from 1950 to 1999, particularly in calcium, potassium, riboflavin, iron, and ascorbic acid content.[33]

Many studies have found that in the last 50 years fruits and vegetables have lost large percentages of their nutrients. So while today's mothers still try to get their children to eat their vegetables, it's getting to the point where it matters very little how many fruits and vegetables we eat. In fact, some experts are arguing that produce is essentially becoming like junk food because it no longer can absorb the necessary nutrients from our depleted soil.

Highlighting the severity of the issue. For example, a 2009 study published in the *Journal of HortScience* found that people also think fruits and vegetables taste worse today than they did in past generations. The researchers who conducted the study more importantly found that the average vegetable found in grocery stores today has between 5 percent and 40 percent fewer minerals than those from 50 years ago. Farmers also harvest fruits and vegetables prematurely to get them to the markets faster, which further saps nutrients from the crops, because they have less time to absorb what's left of the already-depleted nutrients from the soil.

It should not be surprising that you have to eat eight oranges today to obtain the same amount of Vitamin C your grandparents received from a single orange. As you can clearly see, minerals are continuing to vanish from our soil. What is causing this dramatic decrease? Scientists all over the world have offered explanations, from acid rain to chemical fertilization and the use of herbicides and pesticides. The answer may be a combination of all of these entities and other factors.

The use of chemicals in farming prevents crops from up taking (absorbing) even the tiny amounts of micronutrients (called trace minerals) that are now left in our soil. It's also important to note that it's not only that macro minerals, trace minerals, and ultratrace elements are vanishing from our soil, but also the fact that herbicides and pesticides greatly reduce a plant's ability to absorb these minerals.

Bacteria Assist a Plant's Ability to Absorb Minerals

"Soil is a living material," observed Professor John Crawford, a University of Sydney expert in sustainable agriculture. "If you hold a handful of soil, there will be more microorganisms in there than the number of people who have ever lived on the planet. Microbes need carbon for food, but carbon is being lost from the soil in a number of ways."

"Crop breeding is exacerbating this situation," continued Professor Crawford, in an interview with the World Economic Forum. "Modern wheat varieties, for example, have half the micronutrients of older strains, and it's pretty much the same for fruit and vegetables. The focus has been on breeding high-yield crops that can survive on degraded soil, so it's hardly surprising that 60 percent of the world's population is deficient in nutrients. If it's not in the soil, it's not in our food."[34]

All of the organisms living in this ecosystem need many different types of minerals to exist so they can play their part in the soil's ecosystem. These include macro minerals and other mineral nutrients (trace minerals, ultratrace minerals, and trace elements).

Minerals are a critical part of the role plants can play in maximizing our wellness potential.

There are bacteria whose role is to convert these mineral elements into a chemical form so that plants can use them. Unfortunately, the use of certain fertilizers can gradually change the soil's pH towards a more acidic condition in which these bacteria are unable to live. Thus, the bacteria are not able to perform their function to allow plants to absorb these extremely low levels of remaining minerals.

Nitrogen fertilizers "adversely affect the accumulation of vitamin C in various vegetable crops such as lettuce, kale, and Brussels-sprouts," noted a study in the science journal *Plant and Soil*. Vitamin C levels are reduced by more than 25 percent when nitrogen fertilizers are used on crops. Phosphorus fertilizers exact similar nutrient reductions on a wide variety of crops.[35]

What Are What We Call the "Mineral Suites"?

In our nutritional program these are major macronutrients in the category of macro minerals such as potassium, calcium, magnesium, and sulfur); a second level of micronutrients in the categories of trace minerals like iron, copper, and zinc, and the ultra-trace minerals that are elements found in extremely small quantities in our bodies, such as boron, nickel, silicon, vanadium, arsenic, and fluoride. Both the major macro minerals and trace and ultra-trace minerals are essential inorganic elements that are required in small amounts (less than 100 milligrams) for the normal physiologic processes of the body. We require ionic trace minerals and ultra-trace elements to support natural detoxification and to speed up the antioxidant capabilities in the human body.

Selenium is a micronutrient not essential for crops, but essential to humans consuming the crop foods.[35] Major macro minerals and micronutrient trace minerals are essential inorganic elements that are required in small amounts (less than 100 milligrams) for the normal physiologic processes of the body.

For example, selenium is needed for the production of glutathione peroxidase, which is an enzyme that protects the body from oxidative damage. It is a very important natural molecule in the body that is a toxin hunter. It pulls toxins apart and makes them water soluble so they can then be processed by the liver and the kidneys. Is such an important element to a natural ability of the body to detoxify itself.

Zinc, another micronutrient, is essential for many enzymes. Cobalt, a trace element, is part of vitamin B12, as well as the vehicle to efficiently open cells to receive and process nutrients.

Minerals of all kinds support the majority of muscle functions in the human body and are one of the key components of most body processes. While performing so many functions in the body, trace minerals also help eliminate our cravings for sugar and carbohydrates. These little powerhouses that make up the essential categories of minerals we need have been called the spark plugs of life, so when they are lacking in the foods we eat, our ability to live life to the fullest is hindered. Imagine how your car would run if just one spark plug was not working. Ultimately, our human potential is dependent upon having sufficient trace minerals in our diet.

We must constantly keep in mind that today, even if a food source is organically based, it may not contain the proper amount of nutrients, vitamins, and categories of minerals required for optimal health. Therefore, we must supplement to ensure that our bodies natural detoxification system receives all the nutrients essential for optimal functioning to deal with today's onslaught of toxic exposure.

Since toxins diminish absorption, we will continue to have the problem of nutritional depletion in spite of the foods and additional nutrients we consume if we don't rid of the many toxins we are exposed to. Once we understand that this problem exists, it can be our goal to make healthy lifestyle modifications that include healthier food choices, supplementation, exercise, and stress reduction.

The Problem: Uptake of Minerals

Using herbicides and pesticides greatly reduces the uptake of trace minerals by the plants from the soil. As pointed out earlier, plants also need fungi in the soil in order to uptake minerals. This occurs through a process that is called mycorrhiza (this comes from Greek, meaning mushroom and root). The way it works is that plant roots have tiny little hairs, and little threads called mycelia penetrate the hairs of the fungi.

Unbelievably, these fungi connections can cover several acres, and are what allows carbohydrates to be absorbed from the plant roots. Without the fungi to break down minerals, the plants would not be able to absorb the minerals and carbohydrates from the soil, including critically important macro minerals, trace minerals, and ultra-trace minerals.[36]

Plants are susceptible to various fungal diseases. Therefore, these fungal diseases have the adverse effect of decreasing crop yields, causing the farmers to spray chemical fungicides to combat the disease, which sets in motion another vicious cycle of soil degradation. These fungal spays can destroy mycorrhiza fungi. This causes a dilemma because now the plants have less ability to absorb the minerals. The use of insecticides can further reduce the uptake (absorption) of macro minerals because they are destroying enzymes that contain choline, which is an essential component for the absorption of magnesium.

Further Nutrient Losses through Processing and Cooking

On top of crop nutrient losses as a result of mineral depleted soils, processing practices for fruits and vegetables, added to our cooking practices, further reduces the amount of nutrients available for absorption by the human body. Here are just a few examples of how that happens:

- Approximately two-thirds of the original vitamin C in fresh peas is lost during processing.[37]

- Processing potatoes almost totally eradicates ascorbic acid.[38]

- Cooking, especially microwaving food, considerably affects the health-promoting compounds of Brassica vegetables like broccoli, Brussels sprouts, cabbage, cauliflower, and kale. Specifically, it depletes minerals and vitamin C. Boiling and steaming also causes significant vitamin losses in broccoli, in fact you lose 34 percent by boiling and 22 percent by steaming.[39]

ORGANIC VERSUS NON-ORGANIC: A DEBATE OVER NUTRIENT LEVELS

Many people see buying organic fruits and vegetables as the answer to nutrient depletion (and pesticide health concerns). But is that really the answer to our problem of mineral depletion in soils? Whether organic foods contain more nutrients than conventionally farmed crops is a matter of ongoing debate among nutritionists and food scientists. Studies have come down on both sides of the issue. For example, in 2012 a review of 223 studies, published in the *Annals of Internal Medicine*, concluded that there isn't strong evidence to believe that organic foods are significantly more nutritious than conventional foods.[40] Then, two years later, the *British Journal of Nutrition* published an even larger review of 343 studies that found just the opposite. Each of these scientific literature reviews was a meta-analysis, meaning the findings from dozens of different studies were analyzed and compared to reach conclusions about the consensus of opinion.[41]

There was one major difference in approach between the two study reviews: the first one, in 2012, included not only a comparison of organic and non-organic vegetables but also meats, poultry, milk, and eggs. By contrast, the second analysis focused solely on vegetable crop foods. That difference in scope may account for the varying conclusions, though it's important to note that mineral levels between organic and non-organic were relatively the same (except for phosphorus) between both growing techniques. Phosphorus levels were higher in non-organic crops, probably due to the use of phosphorus fertilizers.

Annals of Internal Medicine, Primary 2012 Findings:

"The published literature lacks strong evidence that organic foods are significantly more nutritious than conventional foods."

"The risk for contamination with detectable pesticide residues was 30 percent lower among organic than conventional produce."[42]

British Journal of Nutrition, Primary 2014 Findings:

"The concentrations of a range of antioxidants such as polyphenolics were found to be substantially higher in organic crops."

"The frequency of occurrence of pesticide residues was found to be four times higher in conventional crops," compared to organic crops.

"Significant differences were also detected for mineral and vitamin compounds" in organic crops, compared to conventional.[43]

Then, an article in the *Journal of the Science of Food and Agriculture* claimed:

"There is little evidence that organic and conventional foods differ in respect to the concentrations of the various micronutrients (vitamins, minerals and trace elements)"[44]

The Reason for Organic Produce
Pesticide Contamination

An important clue as to why organically grown crops still contain measureable amounts of pesticides came in the January/February 2006 issue of the *Journal of Environmental Quality*, which published a study showing how pesticides that were spread on croplands and orchards up to a century ago still contaminate the top ten inches of soils where they were used. When farmland or orchards undergo redevelopment, or when soil erosion occurs, the old persistent chemical toxins are released from the soils and migrate into the nearest sources of water, particularly irrigation water. Our lesson from this finding is that past agricultural practices will continue to affect humans and animal life for generations to come.

Even organic crops, because they are mostly grown in nutrient-depleted soils that previously hosted chemical intervention applications, aren't as nutrient rich as they would have been a century ago. Also keep in mind that acid rain, one of the unheralded contributors to the depletion of minerals in soils, doesn't distinguish between organic or non-organic croplands when it falls from the sky. A number of studies discounted organic soils as containing higher minerals and micronutrients than non-organic croplands. A meta-analysis in the *British Journal of Nutrition* argued, "This study does not support the belief that organically grown foodstuffs generally contain more major and trace elements than conventionally grown foodstuffs."

But keep in mind that while organic farming is less toxic, it is a myth that they are nutritionally very different. The organic food farmers do use natural herbicides and pesticides, but there is cross contamination from chemicals blowing from other fields over the soil. The major advantage is that they do not use growth hormones and antibiotics for their livestock.

ESSENTIAL NUTRIENTS AND WHY WE NEED THEM

An essential nutrient is one that is required for normal physiological function; it must be obtained from a dietary source. A total of 23 mineral elements from the soil have been identified as essential in humans, according to *The Handbook of Essential Mineral Elements*, a book of mineral references. Here they are in alphabetical order:

• Arsenic	• Iodine	• Nickel
• Boron	• Iron	• Phosphorus
• Calcium	• Lead	• Potassium
• Chloride	• Lithium	• Selenium
• Chromium	• Magnesium	• Silicon
• Cobalt	• Manganese	• Sodium
• Copper	• Molybdenum	• Vanadium
• Fluoride		• Zinc

Nutritionists also generally identify 13 vitamins as being essential for optimal human body function: Vitamins A, C, D, E, K, and B vitamins (riboflavin, niacin, thiamine, folate, B12, B6, pantothenic acid, and biotin).

Being deficient in the spark plugs of life—nutrients—affects all enzyme reactions in the human body. That is critically important to health and the prevention of disease. The simple definition of a dietary deficiency is a lack of nutrients that the body needs to function properly. These nutrients, including trace elements, minerals, and vitamins, are required for a fully functioning body. Health problems become more serious when there is a deficit in one or more of these micro-nutritional elements.

The Journal of Nutrition Health and Aging listed the micronutrient needs of the human body, along with some of the health disorders caused by their deficiencies. For example:

- Copper deficiency has been linked to Alzheimer's disease.

- Iodine deficiency disrupts metabolism in brain cells.

- Iron deficiency is found in children with attention-deficit/hyperactivity disorder.

- Magnesium is linked to proper functioning of all major body metabolisms.

- Manganese and zinc participate in enzymatic mechanisms that protect the body against free radicals and toxic derivatives of oxygen; zinc deficiency also causes metabolic disturbances.

- Vitamin B12 deficiencies affect the brain and behavior in people of all ages, but particularly children.

- Trace element deficiencies are connected to brain diseases, mental under-development in children, infirmities of aging, and so on.[45]

Food is one of the most powerful medicines available, but it is now being replaced by so-called "super foods," which despite all the marketing about their health benefits still don't contain the high levels of nutrients we need. Let's be clear: Nutritional deficiency is a much bigger problem than simply being hungry. The deficiencies in micronutrients alone are costing us our health and our futures. Experts estimate the body requires several dozen essential nutrients, and studies reveal that many are now lacking in our fresh fruits and vegetables. There we have identified another connection within the TDOS Syndrome, as a contributing co-factor for triggering stress and weight gain.

I believe there are two types of hunger. **Psychological hunger** is not caused by an actual, physical pain nor a need for food to survive. Psychological hunger is caused by a desire to eat either out of habit, because you see good food around you, because you are emotional or upset, or because it tastes good and is "fun." **Physical Hunger** on the other hand is satisfied when signals from the brain, GI tract, and hormonal system receive the required nutrients to turn off the hunger.

Processed food created by our Food Industry combine fat, salt, and sugar to in a manner that triggers psychological hunger, craving, and overeating.

—NICHOLAS MESSINA, MD

HOW COMMON ARE NUTRIENT DEFICIENCIES?

"Widespread global micronutrient deficiencies exist," warned a 2015 study in the science journal *Annals of Nutrition and Metabolism*. "Pregnant women and their children under 5 years are at the highest risk. Iron, iodine, folate, vitamin A, and zinc deficiencies are the most widespread micronutrient deficiencies and all are common contributors to poor growth, intellectual impairments, perinatal complications, and increased risk of morbidity and mortality."

After pointing out how adequate zinc is necessary for optimal immune system function, folate is essential to DNA synthesis and repair, and vitamin A for eye health, the authors of this study note the deficiencies and issue this alarm: "Perhaps of greatest concern is the cycle of micronutrient deficiencies that persists over generations and the intergenerational consequences of micronutrient deficiencies that we are only beginning to understand."[46]

"Today, there are over 3.7 billion iron-deficient individuals and about 1 billion people that are at risk of developing iodine deficiency disorders," estimated Ross M. Welch, a soil and nutrition scientist with the United States Department of Agriculture, in a 2002 study for the science journal *Plant and Soil*. "There are over 200 million people that are vitamin A deficient, {and millions more} deficient in zinc, selenium, vitamin C, vitamin D, and folic acid."[47]

Studies targeting specific groups of people, testing nutrient absorption levels, have reached similar conclusions. More than 300 female college students gave blood samples in a 2014 study, examining biomarkers for iron, vitamin B12, folate, selenium, zinc, and copper. Serious micronutrient deficiencies were measured in most of the students for iron, B12, copper, and selenium.[48]

A 2015 study review of experiments targeting adults 65 years and older found six nutrients "of possible public health concern" that were found to be inadequate: vitamin D, thiamin, riboflavin, calcium, magnesium, and selenium.[49]

"Nutrient deficiencies occur {even in populations eating} a balanced and varied diet," observed a 2014 study in *Nutrition Journal*, "including in populations with bountiful food supplies and the means to procure nutrient-rich foods. For example, the typical American diet bears little resemblance to what experts recommend for fruit, vegetables, and whole grains. With time, deficiencies in one or more micronutrients may lead to serious health issues."[50]

MISCONCEPTIONS REGARDING
THE STATE OF NUTRITION

Let's clarify some misconceptions about the overall state of nutrition and where the essential nutrients really originate. Taking a trip to the local grocery store will only confuse those who haven't taken the time to find the truth. Walking down the aisles, we see claims for fortified foods, reduced fat, diet, and, the big one these days, organic. Ultimately, these catch phrases are nothing more than brilliant marketing.

If all this advertising for these products were true, we would not be struggling with nutritional deficiency. There are misunderstandings about these slogans, including use of the word "organic." While organic foods, especially produce, are somewhat better for you in some ways, they are still nutritionally inadequate, as we mentioned earlier. Nutritional deficiency (or insufficiency) in our bodies starts with nutritionally bankrupt food. And nutritionally bankrupt food grows out of nutritionally bankrupt soil.

To give you an illustration, if organic plants are grown in the same dirt as non-organic plants, with the only difference being the lack of pesticides and herbicides in the organic fields, does this increase the nutritional value of the organic plant? No. Just because it's organic doesn't necessarily mean the nutritional density is any higher than other produce, given the overall condition of our soils.

While we do not want to discourage people from eating organic foods, we want people to understand that the goal should be to get what is possible from the best food sources available and then learn to supplement the nutrients that are not available from your sources.

Remember, the body is mainly concerned about nutrients and the lack thereof—not calories, per se. Eating organic foods will not completely satisfy the body's hunger for sustenance because the nutrients (like trace minerals) are still missing from our food. Our bodies desperately crave more nutrients in the form of major minerals (macro minerals), micronutrient minerals (trace minerals) and ultra-trace elements. The body requires, in some cases, minute almost microscopic amounts of them for good health.

NUTRIENT DECLINES ALSO AFFECT ORGANIC FOODS

So where does nutrition come from? Nutritionists agree that it originates in a balanced diet—but that "balanced diet" is composed of a wide variety of foods. All experts agree that an essential nutrient is a nutrient that the body cannot synthesize on its own—or not to an adequate amount—and must be provided by the diet. These nutrients are necessary for the body to function properly. The six essential nutrients include carbohydrates, protein, fat, vitamins, minerals and water.

What experts cannot agree on are the proper sources and individual amounts of these six essential nutrients needed for optimal functioning. In today's fast paced, convenience-driven world, the majority of the population is not receiving the proper amounts or the proper combinations of these nutrients on a daily basis.

Dr. Arden Andersen, who has degrees in both medicine and agriculture, addressed the lack of nutrients and where this nutritional deficiency stems from in a 2008 article "The Root of Good Nutrition." Dr. Andersen has extensive experience not only as a physician but also as a consultant in the food production industry and as a surgeon in the armed forces. He has also conducted numerous studies on crop and animal management. According to Dr. Andersen's research, the nutrient content of foods today, compared to half a century ago, ranges from 15 to 75 percent less.[51]

This decline includes foods that are labeled organic. The fact of the matter is that the food itself today is significantly deficient in nutrient density due to the poor agricultural practices of the farmers who grow the food, including much of the "certified organic" food. When we look back over the decades, we see more clearly how agriculture has really dropped the ball relative to nutrition in the soil and getting that nutrition into the plant to supplement the food we eat.

An increase in disease today may be directly attributable to deficiencies in the supply of trace minerals in our diets. These deficiencies do not stem from a lack of available food (quantity). Rather, they stem from the lack of good quality food and a failure to consume all essential nutrients on a daily basis.

MOST VITAMIN AND MINERAL SUPPLEMENTS FALL SHORT

The main job of micro minerals is to "hold the house together." Micro minerals, in a sense, are akin to the numerous tiny nails, nuts, and bolts that hold a house together. If all of these are slowly removed and never replaced, the house will begin to sag and eventually fall apart. The same is true with these trace minerals, which are among the smallest building blocks in our bodies.

Micronutrient minerals are important in the proper functioning of enzyme systems, nerve conduction and muscle function, assisting with transfer of nourishment into cells, providing the framework for tissues, and regulation of organ functions. These "behind the scenes" functions are impossible without a constant, adequate supply of micro minerals.

Walk into any health food store or drugstore and you will find a boggling assortment of nutritional supplements. But when you examine the ingredients, there isn't enough focus on the trace mineral content. Most multivitamin and mineral supplements fall short because they do not contain enough well-rounded categories of minerals. Another problem with some supplements is that they are hard for the body to absorb. The molecular content of nutrients within the supplements can be too large for the body to break down. A key point to remember is that it's not about quantity; it's about absorbability.

Returning to Dr. Arden Anderson's point earlier, the problem starts beneath our feet, in the actual soil used to produce our food. We are living in a nutritionally deficient world. Over the last 60 years, iron levels in spinach have dropped over 4,300 percent, according to a study conducted at Cornell University.[52]

Study after study reveals that our food is headed toward nutritional bankruptcy as our soil continues to be under siege from herbicides, pesticides, and over farming. These persistent attacks on the soil (where it all begins) and this escalation of nutrition loss affects everything, from broccoli to Brussels sprouts, from cauliflower to spinach.

RECEIVING NECESSARY AMOUNTS OF NUTRIENTS

The nutrition deficiency solution seems, on the face of it, rather easy: Find a source, or create your own recipe, for nutrient-dense food. But think about what that really means. Even for the hungriest among us, it seems impossible to sit down and eat 30 bowls of spinach. And that just matches the nutritional levels measured in 1973. Those 30 bowls of spinach would only satisfy the necessary iron levels for one day.

Research reveals that most Americans are deficient in one or more of the essential nutrients. This not only means they are receiving less than they need for optimal health but that they are receiving less than the minimum amount of nutrients necessary to prevent deficiency states. It means Americans are receiving less than the *minimum amount* of nutrients necessary to prevent deficiency diseases.

Now that irrefutable evidence exists that Americans are not receiving adequate nutrition and that this deficiency helps produce a disease state within the body, what are the food companies doing to help solve this major problem? They are not addressing this cataclysmic problem. These companies are, in fact, taking food in the opposite direction from where it needs to be.

PROCESSED FOOD CHEMISTRY RESEMBLES ADDICTIVE DRUGS

It's clear that the ramifications of using excessive salt, sugar, and fat are changing our entire nutritional landscape. Not only are we facing a major nutritional crisis but also the American diet is now even more distorted in favor of profit versus health considerations. By concentrating fat, salt, and sugar in products formulated for maximum "bliss," the "Big Food" industry has spent almost a century warping the American diet into high calorie, low nutrition "food products" whose consumption pattern has been mirrored by the calamitous rise in obesity.

The majority of food manufacturers have only one goal in mind, and it's not to solve the overweight epidemic or create a healthier population. Their main goal is to maximize profit, which is what corporations are designed to do. Food manufacturers have invented food categories to improve their bottom lines. They have played off two major ideas. First, to generate return customers, ingredients are manipulated to form addictive qualities to these foods. The second idea coincides with the rapid pace of our society. We have less time to cook traditional meals, thus, we rely on convenient food "products," such as one-minute macaroni and pre-packaged lunch trays.

These convenience foods have several things in common. They are highly processed, with cheap ingredients designed to satisfy us for a short time without slowing down our day. What these food companies are doing is absolutely immoral. They have teams of scientists investigating how to manipulate foods to play tricks on the brain. By researching the pleasure centers in the brain and concocting the perfect blend of sugar, salt, and fat, these labs are discovering how to maximize profits by playing off that old catch phrase, "No one can eat just one." When a person can't just eat one, profit margins become as fat as our waistlines.

The fight against processed foods is, in many ways, comparable to the massive "war on drugs" in this country. The government has sent millions of people to jail for manufacturing and selling illegal drugs that control people by influencing the pleasure centers in the brain, causing addiction. Some of these processed foods mimic the levels of addiction caused by drugs. Using the same brain chemistry that is manipulated by drugs, food scientists have found ways to duplicate the sensations a drug user experiences. Instead of drugs, they use manufactured, nutrient-bereft food chemical products.

According to Michael Moss's research in his book *Sugar, Salt and Fat*, there are no regulations as to the amount of sugar used in foods, while proof abounds that the body can sustain major damage when abusing sugar, salt, and fat. It can be argued that these "bliss point" foods are as dangerous as drugs. Some of these foods can help stimulate disease states in the body, leading to any number of health problems—including death.

The first step is to become aware of the ramifications of our nutritional deficiency and the sinister use of salt, sugar, and fat. There is no question that these ingredients have been used to disguise processed food's nutritional bankruptcy. In using toxic amounts of salt, sugar, and fat, we have distorted our taste buds. The American palate is so accustomed to the overuse of these ingredients that unrefined, unprocessed food no longer tastes "normal."

Melanie Warner, a recent guest on my TV show *The New Health Conversation* and former business reporter for *The New York Times*, was sharing research results from her book *Pandora's Lunch Box*. This is an amazing investigative journey into the secret world of processed foods. She pointed out that companies now have food engineers creating chemicals that mimic food.

About 70 percent of the calories we eat are from packaged foods and fast food, according to Warner, and our diets have changed more during the last century than they have in the last 10,000 years. In her book, she offers an inside look at the food manufacturing industry and explains why food processing plays such a major role in our nation's rapidly-expanding waistlines and the fact that half of Americans suffer from at least one chronic disease related to their diet.

Only time can heal our wounded taste buds. But how can they recover when there is no escape from the high-calorie, low-nutrient industrialized food culture? It has been said that if a product can be sweetened, it has been over sweetened; if there is a need for a pinch of salt, chances are that more than a handful gets added.

WE OVEREAT BECAUSE WE'RE ADDICTS

We are the most overfed and yet undernourished country in the world. The primary reason we overeat is a result of the mass consumption of empty calories filled with the combination of salt, sugar, and fat, which leads to craving and psychological hunger. There is no substance in these calories to satisfy the body's need for nutrition. When the body receives nutritionally-dense calories, physical hunger dissipates. Without that density, physical hunger intensifies. A great example of the difference between an empty calorie and a nutritionally dense one is like comparing a balloon filled with air to one filled with water. The body would need far fewer water balloons to feel full.

All these findings call for a new health conversation. If we continue to allow food companies to play to our distorted taste buds, the consequences of nutritional deficiency will be devastating. There may be no recovery if we don't act now. This conversation is the only strategy to save us from our own self-destructive ignorance. Using food to satiate ourselves is not enough. We need to fill our bodies with the proper nutrients and that begins with public education.

No human being today can consume the amount of fruits and vegetables required for optimum health, because our stomachs are not large enough. The government's term, RDA (Recommended Daily Allowance), is a guideline for people to ensure they receive adequate vitamins and minerals every day. In another lifetime, this guideline may have been of some value. The problem is that this chart does not take into consideration the depletion of vitamins and minerals in our foods. The RDA guidelines are laid out for people with generally good health, minimal stress, and little to no exposure to toxins (which is no one).

In medical school, doctors receive very little education on diet and nutrition. It is up to each physician to do his or her own research on the effects of poor nutrition. When physicians test patients' cholesterol levels and blood pressure, usually their solutions are pharmaceutically based. Either that or patients are advised to change dietary habits and omit certain foods. Discussions about introducing macro and micro-nutrients are infrequent in those conversations, possibly because there is little evidence to support the overstated claims made on supplement labels.

Many doctors still buy into two outdated major schools of thought. The first is that the body can get all its nourishment, including vitamins and minerals, from food alone. The second belief is that as long as a person fits into the proper "weight category," there should be no concern about malnutrition in these patients.

—NICHOLAS MESSINA, MD

EVEN POPULAR DIET PLANS ARE NUTRITIONALLY DEFICIENT

Counting calories is not the answer if, at the same time, you ignore the nutrient density of the calories you are consuming. Unless the calorie is nutrient dense, you push the body into starvation mode because of the lack of nutrition. This is what so infuriates us as authors. Many popular diet programs keep talking about reducing calories by offering you low-calorie processed foods, but they do not address the nutritional insufficiency of the reduced caloric food they recommend eating. Unless you make up for the nutritional deficiency, you are going to hurt your body in the long run.

Remember, the body only cares about nutrients that get absorbed. The calorie is just a measurement, and counting calories while ignoring nutritional deficiency appears to be a flawed strategy in the long run. Period.

Nutritionally dense foods offer a new way of thinking. We call these new ways of thinking about nutrition new nutritional approaches. Instead of counting calories we should be making every calorie count, based on the nutritional density of the calories we are consuming.

The *Journal of the International Society of Sports Nutrition* decided to test whether three of the most popular diet plans were deficient in micronutrient needs for the human body. It was a damning and revealing study that received too little attention in the mainstream media. Several of the most popular diet plans were evaluated.

In the first diet analyzed, it was estimated that 20,500 calories needed to be consumed daily to meet the micronutrient requirements. Basically that is between five and ten times the calories needed to maintain a healthy weight. In another one of these popular diets, the study estimated that you would need to consume 18,800 calories a day and, on another popular diet, the dieters would have to consume a staggering 37,500 calories a day! Again, this was just to meet the minimum micronutrient sufficiency based on the daily RDI (recommended daily intake).

This 2010 study found that if you were to follow the 2011 food pyramid for healthy eating, in order to hit the new "recommended daily intake" (RDI) for vitamins and minerals, you would need to consume between 3,500 to 5,500 calories each day. The study author concluded: "These findings are significant and indicate that an individual following a popular diet plan as suggested with food alone, has a high likelihood of becoming micronutrient deficient; a state shown to be scientifically linked to an increased risk for many dangerous and debilitating health conditions and diseases."[53]

Keep in mind that the term RDI refers to a specific calculation of essential vitamins and minerals the body needs. The RDI is not the daily optimal amount of essential nutrients the body needs—it is more of a baseline measure of what is needed to prevent malnutrition. The RDI is more extensive, listing basic vitamins and minerals as well as micronutrients. It is a step in the right direction, but it can also be misleading when taken out of context. It is also important to restate that it is merely a baseline, not necessarily what the body actually needs.

It seems clear based on the most conservative evidence that it is nearly impossible to consume enough food to meet our basic nutritional needs every day. It's implausible for most people to even come close to hitting the minimum requirements based purely on the amount of food needed to reach the RDI. We need a drastic change in how and what we eat. It clearly starts in the earth itself. There needs to be a re-education about the degradation of our food supply. We have an abundance of readily available food but none of it is fit to nourish our bodies. What precedent are we setting for our young people?

NUTRIENT DEFICIENCY STARTS EARLY IN LIFE

Turn on the television and tune into any kids' channel. You'll see commercials aimed at persuading children to eat anything from highly processed "lunchables" to cookie-flavored cereals. Using cartoon characters and placing toys in the box is only the first step in selling our youth on a nutritionally deficient lifestyle. Once these cereals are consumed, the industrialized food producers' goal is to find the same "bliss point" in our kids, to hook them from the very beginning. By marketing to youngsters, parents are often pushed by their children into buying these colorful boxes of "dead flakes in a cardboard coffin," and the deficiency spiral begins. Parents buy these ridiculous products masquerading as food, feed it to their kids, and then wonder why their children are overweight and prone to illness.

The statistics are frightening. As mentioned earlier, statistics estimate that one in three babies born in the US today will develop diabetes in his or her lifetime. Ten years from now, up to 50 percent of children are likely to be overweight. It doesn't take much research to understand that proper nutrition is absolutely vital for growing kids. Who is teaching these kids about nutrition? Is it the parents or is it the marketing machine behind Saturday morning cartoons? It certainly seems to be a combination of the two.

Equally important, adequate nutrition is critical for growing fetuses. Nutritional education should begin *before* a baby is born. We are conditioning our next generation in the womb. It is well accepted in medical circles that a pregnant woman, deficient in nutrients, can contribute to stunting the growth and development of an unborn child. As these children grow and become adults, they are more susceptible to becoming overweight, as well as possibly suffering from chronic diseases, including diabetes and hypertension. Nutritional deficiency is a major crisis.

TDOS SYNDROME CO-FACTORS MAGNIFY THE PROBLEMS

Now that it's apparent how we are nutritionally starving, we need to return to the toxicity factor. Nutritional deficiency plays a major role in the buildup of toxicity in the body. The good news is that the body is capable of naturally detoxifying itself of impurities and toxins. The bad news is that without a massive amount of nutrients, the body becomes sluggish and less effective at purifying itself, thus allowing toxins to collect in dangerous quantities.

The combination of toxicity and nutritional deficiency opens the floodgates to the third co-factor, the overweight epidemic. Without the proper amount of nutrients needed to fuel the body's natural toxin hunters, and to support the body's detoxification mechanism, toxins are allowed to roam free. We already know some of the devastating effects these toxins have in the body. If the body can't naturally detoxify itself, obesogens, or additional fat cells, are produced to protect the body's vital organs, thus creating weight gain and obesity. The inner connectivity of these co-factors only raises the stakes in this harmful health game.

Unfortunately, there are no longer just one or two solutions that will allow us to dig our way out of these unhealthy lifestyles. Exercise and healthy eating are the two leading paths to maintaining optimum health, but they are no longer sufficient. Working out is more critical than ever, but without the missing nutrition the body requires, it no longer has a fraction of the same benefits.

In March 2006 the United Nations recognized a new kind of malnutrition—a multiple micronutrient depletion. According to Catherine Bertini, Chair of the United Nations Standing Committee on Nutrition, those who are overweight are just as malnourished as those who are starving. We are now back to a familiar theme: It's not the quantity of food that is at issue; it's the quality. If you think that food will ever be sufficient, when it lacks all of these minerals, think again.

Michael Pollan, author of the bestselling books *The Omnivore's Dilemma* and *In Defense of Food*, said it best when he pointed out that you are not only what you eat but, "You are what it eats too. If our beef is loaded with hormones that are designed to cause artificial weight gain, and we eat said beef . . . Wouldn't we be likely to gain unnatural amounts of weight too?"

Due to the prevalence of pesticides, herbicides, and antibiotics in food, very little of what humans eat can be fully broken down by the body. Instead, these toxic elements are being stored in our bodies as fat, and ultimately these toxins in fat contribute to the overall degeneration of human health, as the next section of this book will illuminate.

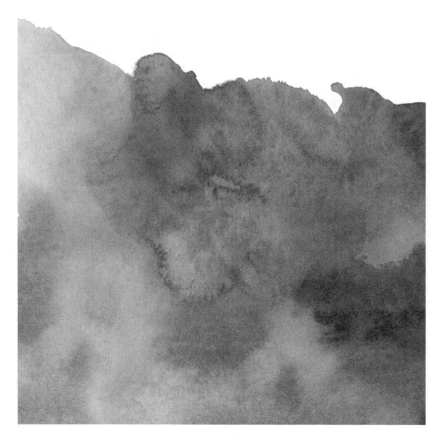

PART THREE

Co-Factor O—**Overweight**

Co-Factor O—Overweight

What We Don't Know About Weight Is Hurting Us

My mother, Grace, was morbidly obese most of her life. For all the years she was on this earth, I think she tried every fad diet that existed. Yet, in spite of all those diets, fads, and gimmicks, I never knew my mom to be thin—or healthy.

One particularly hot, muggy day in July 2000 in Biddeford, Maine, I was walking alone down a long hallway in a hospital where I had gone when I was suddenly called to see my mother. The only sounds I could hear were the echoes of my footsteps, and the slow mechanical breathing of a respirator at the end of the hall. I came to a doorway and looked in. There, to my surprise, lay my mother. She had suffered a massive heart attack and stroke. Although she hung on for a few days, it was too late. No second chance at health . . . or life. No do-over. No escaping the years of abuse her body had endured, under the tremendous weight she carried around.

Six months before she died, my mother said something that stays with me after all these years. She said, "Peter, you know I have one wish in my life that I have never achieved."

"What's that, mom?"

"It is the wish that when I die, I would die thin," she said.

Her words continue to haunt me every time I appear on stage to speak with people about health, even though I've conducted more than 1,000 of these lectures around the world. I believe that if I had known then, what I now know about the TDOS Syndrome, maybe my mom might still be alive.

Many of us, like my mother, struggle with additional weight, and the statistics reveal that this is only getting worse. But we will never reverse this problem if we remain stuck on calorie counting instead of acknowledging the huge role that toxins and nutritional deficiencies play both in our weight gain and in our inability to lose that weight. Obesogens are real and they trigger our weight gain—along with a host of other harmful diseases. Traditional diets are not the answer. In fact, many low-calorie diets cause stress, which actually leads to weight gain instead of weight loss. This chapter will arm you with the information you need to better understand the real cause of overweight and obesity.

WE FACE A SERIOUS GLOBAL WEIGHT PROBLEM

The rising trend of seeing people excessively overweight is an epidemic. It has risen steadily in the United States during the past 150 years and has accelerated dramatically in the past few decades. Obesity is rising worldwide, including an alarming increase among developing countries. Clearly, the current strategies to stem this tide by the medical and scientific communities have been ineffective. We are losing the battle against people becoming disproportionately overweight, and we must rethink our approach before we lose the war.

Statistics paint a grim and numbing picture of the breadth and gravity of the situation humanity faces:

Americans, on average, have become the fattest people on the planet. In 1990, not one of the 50 states registered more than 15 percent of its population as being overweight or obese; just 20 years later, at least 18 states reported more than 30 percent of its population as overweight or obese.[54]

Excess weight may have already become a national security issue for the US armed forces. Some 27 percent of young people enrolling in our military programs are rejected because of weight problems.[55]

If current trends continue, healthcare experts predict that by 2030, at least 86 percent of US adults will be overweight or obese. That will burden the economy with nearly $1 trillion in additional health-care costs.[56]

This is not just a big problem for America. It is a worldwide phenomenon.

In China, the numbers of children and adolescents who are obese grew from just 1 percent of those under 19 years of age in 1985, to more than 17 percent of boys and 9 percent of girls by 2014, the fastest rate of obesity growth ever recorded on the planet.[57]

From 1975 to 2014, global obesity in men tripled, and obesity in women more than doubled, based on statistics compiled by medical experts writing in the British medical journal *The Lancet.* There are now more obese people on the planet than underweight people.[58]

Of the top 10 leading causes of death, being overweight is a contributing risk factor for five reasons people die prematurely.[59]

As waistlines have ballooned, so have the number of diabetes cases directly attributable to this excess weight: Nearly 10 percent of the world's population now has been diagnosed with either type 1 or type 2 diabetes.

All of these statistics confirm that we absolutely must change our understanding and approach to weight gain if we want to increase our longevity and avoid life-threatening health problems.[60]

The 2016 Global Nutrition Report released on June 14, 2016 is written by more than one hundred independent experts in the field of nutrition. The report stated that 57 of 129 countries in their study have "serious levels" of undernutrition and an increasing problem with obesity. An article by Daisy Meager published on Vice.com on June 15 titled "A New Global Report Says That One Third of People Are Malnourished" states:

> "According to the experts, malnutrition, which the NHS defines as "a serious condition that occurs when a person's diet

doesn't contain the right amount of nutrients," directly affects one in three people and is 'by far the biggest risk factor for the global burden of disease.' . . . But when it comes to the causes of malnutrition, the report found that obesity is becoming a bigger factor. Highlighted particularly in children, the research found that out of the 667 million children under five-years-old worldwide, 50 million 'do not weigh enough for their height' and '41 million are overweight.'"

A NEW DISCOVERY ABOUT WHAT *REALLY* MAKES US FAT

If you think that gaining weight is just about eating too much, absorbing too many calories, and not getting enough exercise—think again! Scientists at the Department of Developmental and Cell Biology, University of California, Irvine, examined the health impact from a category of toxins called endocrine disrupting chemicals (EDCs), and how these toxins influence weight gain, while thwarting attempts to lose weight. It didn't receive much publicity, or medical expert attention, as pioneering medical studies with startling findings go. But it certainly should have, given its profound implications for the future of human health.

"There is an urgent, unmet need to understand the mechanisms underlying how exposure to certain EDCs may predispose our population to be obese," the scientists wrote for their study, published in 2016 by the *American Journal of Obstetrics and Gynecology*.

Though this connection between weight gain and EDC toxins—particularly a subset of EDCs called "obesogens"—had been theorized a few years earlier, the authors of this study took the research to a deeper and unprecedented level of understanding by asking how and why this connection happens. The term "obesogens," referring to environmental chemical molecules that trigger weight gain, was first coined in 2006 by two university scientists writing in the journal *Endocrinology*.

Think of obesogens as metabolic disrupters in the human body, which are skilled at promoting the creation of excess body fat "by altering programming of fat cell development, increasing energy storage in fat tissue, and interfering with neuroendocrine control of appetite," as the study research team explained.

While the dramatic increase in obesity among all age groups is alarming in itself, what alerted the scientists to a thornier problem was "the rise in obesity rates among children under two years of age . . . since it is improbable that children in this age group are consuming more food or exercising less than previous generations."

What became clear to the scientists was that toxic chemical influences from mother to fetus, as the fetus developed in the womb, were programming the children to unnaturally develop excess fat deposits after being born. In other words, many children are being born to become fat, no matter how much they exercise or how healthy they eat.

This finding added a whole new dimension of complicating factors to the problem of weight gain, obesity, and people's failed attempts to lose weight and keep off the excess pounds. This inter-generational genetic relay race, passing on the effects of toxins and nutrient deficiencies and resulting fat storage, is now one emerging aspect of a field of science called "epigenetics." It's the study of how we can inherit changes inflicted on our parent's genes, caused by environmental influences they experience.

"Recent research supports a role for exposure to endocrine-disrupting chemicals (EDCs) in the global obesity epidemic," observed the authors of a study, in a 2015 edition of the science journal *Endocrinology*. "Obesogenic EDCs have the potential to inappropriately stimulate adipogenesis {fat development} and fat storage, influence metabolism and energy balance and increase susceptibility to obesity. Developmental exposure to obesogenic EDCs is proposed to interfere with epigenetic programming of gene regulation, partly by activation of nuclear receptors, thereby influencing the risk of obesity later in life." The conclusion? Obesogens make us fat.[61]

ROUND UP THE UNUSUAL SUSPECTS

To identify the toxic chemical obesogens at the root of this problem, the University of California, Irvine, scientists sifted through dozens of studies over the course of a decade on humans and animal life to assess their accumulated findings. Obesogens turned out to be environmental chemicals that disrupt the human hormonal system in ways that trigger weight gain and, ultimately, a range of diseases starting with type 2 diabetes. These toxins hijack the regulatory systems that humans naturally possess to control body weight. It can also be said that our body's ongoing attempt to protect itself from the constant assault of these chemical toxins results in the production and storage of fat.

Numerous synthetic chemicals emerged as suspected, or documented, culprits and co-conspirators. They include artificial hormones fed to livestock, which become our food sources. They also include plastic pollutants in some food packaging, chemicals added to processed foods, pesticides sprayed on our produce, a marine and agricultural fungicide called tributyltin, phthalates, DDE (a virtually indestructible residue of DDT), and the long list goes on and on. We are not only surrounded by them but also cannot escape them.

These chemicals mimic how human hormones behave, such as the hormone estrogen, and block the actions of other hormones, such as testosterone. These toxins can even alter the functions of our genes, which for many scientists turned out to be the most alarming finding of all.

One of these chemicals, bisphenol A—the building block of hard, polycarbonate plastic, found in food can linings and baby bottles—exerts surprising and strong effects on cells growing in lab dishes. Usually, cells become fibroblasts that make up the body's connective tissue. However, pre-fibroblasts have the potential to become adipocytes, or fat cells. Studies have shown that bisphenol A, and some other industrial compounds, pushed pre-fibroblasts to become fat cells and stimulated the proliferation of existing fat cells.

Biochemist Jerry Heindel, PhD, an expert on endocrine disrupting chemicals for the National Institute for Environmental Health, believes these findings pose a serious and long-term challenge: "The fact that an environmental chemical has the potential to stimulate growth of pre-adipocytes has enormous implications." Research by Heindel and his colleagues indicate that a person's toxic burden can have consequences for three to four generations after the time of exposure.[62]

So the toxin exposure that a pregnant woman receives affects her children, grandchildren, and great grandchildren. This is transgenerational programmed obesity on a monumental scale.

"The implications are profound," wrote the authors of the University of California, Irvine, study I discussed above. "The higher number of fat cells from the beginning of life cannot be reduced by diet, exercise, or even surgery."

That is why, according to the study authors, "up to 87 percent of those who achieve significant weight loss, regain the weight within a few years, supporting the existence of altered metabolic set points."

Considering all this information—the buildup of chemicals, pesticides, and hormones in the body—it's clear that a strong correlation exists between a person's toxic burden and the size of his or her waistline.

Dr. Paula Baillie-Hamilton is a medical doctor and visiting fellow in occupational and environmental health at Stirling University in Scotland. She is also considered to be one of the world's leading authorities on toxic chemicals and their effects on our health. She prophetically wrote, back in 2005: "What appears to be happening is that our natural slimming system is being poisoned by the toxic chemicals we encounter in our everyday lives, and this damage is making it increasingly difficult for our bodies to control their weight. The end result is that we gain weight in the form of fat and not muscle, as chemicals tend to cause muscles to shrink and body fat to accumulate."

This process of toxins transferred into fat is also shortening our lives. In a study conducted in Sweden, it was found that when eight to twelve year olds engaged in a single winter of overeating, the result could be a six-year decrease in lifespan for their grandchildren, because the effects of this overeating were passed on through changes in gene expression, affecting each subsequent generation.[63]

Always keep in mind there is also an entire range of other health impacts from this genetically programmed overeating, from type 2 diabetes to cardiovascular disease. Toxins and nutrient deficiencies truly are programming us to eat ourselves into an early grave, a planet-wide phenomenon that resembles nothing less than a mass extinction event.

THE REAL ENEMY IS TOXINS, NOT CALORIES

If you've ever seen the television programs *The Biggest Loser* and *My 600-lb Life*, then you know how difficult and heart-breaking the process of losing huge amounts of weight can be. Particularly in the case of *The Biggest Loser* contestants, they undergo exhausting and disciplined routines with trainers that involve limiting their calorie intakes and burning a substantial number of calories through vigorous exercise, often for three hours or more a day. While many of the participants in these programs do initially lose considerable amounts of weight after dieting, exercise, or even surgery—sometimes losing hundreds of pounds—the threat always exists for them to regain some, if not most, of that weight.

To determine the extent to which regaining weight actually occurs, a team of researchers writing in the medical journal *Obesity* tracked a group of 14 contestants from *The Biggest Loser* competition, performing diagnostic tests on them six years after their weight loss.

Their body composition was measured and compared when they started the competition, at the 30-week point ending the competition, and again six years later.[64] Losing weight during the competition had dramatically slowed their metabolisms, according to the study, meaning their bodies stopped burning enough calories to maintain a thinner size. The result was that six years after losing the pounds, most had regained much of the original weight. Some are even heavier today than when they started the competition.

Contestant Danny Cahill, a land surveyor who had shed 239 pounds over seven months to win the Season 8 show in 2009, illustrated a typical experience. He dropped from 430 pounds down to 191 pounds, and in his words, "I got my life back. I felt like a million bucks."[65]

But six years after winning the weight- loss competition, Cahill had regained more than 100 pounds, despite continuing to count calories and maintaining an exercise regimen. Researchers in the study attributed his weight regain to a slower metabolism, and to his periodically losing the battle with constant food cravings. Those cravings could be explained by the hormone leptin, an appetite stimulator, whose levels drift up as weight is regained, triggering the urge to eat.

While one key finding of this study has much merit and a universal lesson—the challenge of losing weight and keeping it off is about human biology, not a lack of willpower—the emphasis placed in the study on a slower metabolism as a primary explanation seems short-sighted. It's an explanation very much in need of a larger context for interpretation, given what we know the field of endocrinology has found about the role that obesogens play in promoting weight gain.

This is where the research disconnect occurs. Nowhere in the *Obesity* journal study, nor in *The New York Times* and other news coverage of that study, were important findings about the role of obesogens even mentioned. Not once! The study of *The Biggest Loser* contestants was conducted by metabolism experts at the National Institute of Diabetes and Kidney Diseases, whereas the studies of obesogens were mostly performed by cell biologists in the Department of Pharmaceutical Sciences, University of California, Irvine. Are the experts in metabolism talking to the experts in cell biology and sharing their respective findings about the causes and mechanisms of obesity? Apparently not in this case! Yet, the findings of their studies, as outlined here, may be both compatible and reconcilable.

It's not a stretch, not even for a layman, to see how a slower metabolism after weight loss can be a result of exposure to obesogen chemicals, either as cell programming experienced in the womb before birth or afterwards as a function of daily living contact with endocrine disrupting chemicals in the environment. Obesogens promote obesity by altering metabolic set-points and disrupting appetite controls. These altered metabolisms and inability to control food cravings are exactly what *The Biggest Loser* study found as promoting weight gain in their test subjects.

That experts in divergent fields of medicine aren't fully taking into account each other's research findings is another reason why we wrote this book. Someone needed to assemble all of the elements of the TDOS Syndrome in one place, exposing both the obvious and subtle interconnections and where the "experts" have failed to apply a holistic and synergistic point of view. Given the billions of dollars that Americans spend on weight-loss drugs and diet programs each year, and the toll on mental health that the resulting failures and frustrations they experience brings, we must more clearly understand the reasons why our best efforts at self-control fail, when we are pitted against our own biology and the many unnatural influences on it.

MORE EVIDENCE FOR THE TOXINS-OBESITY LINK

For those of you who prefer abundant scientific evidence, this section has you in mind. In just the past few years, a veritable explosion of research has emerged linking environmental toxins to weight gain, metabolic disorders, and type 2 diabetes. The following examples illustrate both how these persistent organic pollutants trigger weight gain and conversely how weight loss actually increases their levels in our blood.

Persistent Organic Pollutants (POPs) Accelerate Weight Gain

Many human-made chemicals formerly used in agricultural and manufacturing processes have been banned or regulated and are no longer in wide use. Yet, these chemicals are so toxic they remain in the environment and in our food supply, continuing to contaminate us. In the process, these toxins accelerate the development of obesity and pre-diabetes. A good example of a POP is the pesticide DDT, banned in most countries decades ago because of its toxicity, which lives on in the soil in the form of DDE, a virtually indestructible by-product.

Writing in a 2014 issue of *The Journal of Clinical Endocrinology & Metabolism*, a team of scientists from Canada and Norway searched for POPs in a group of 76 obese women of similar ages. Those women with the highest cardio metabolic risk for diabetes, heart disease, or stroke turned out to be the most obese women. These women had the highest number and highest concentrations of 12 POPs stored in their fat. These persistent toxins included dioxins, polychlorinated biphenyls, and organochlorine pesticides, all of which had previously been identified as obesogens and endocrine and metabolic disrupters.[66]

Long-Term Weight Loss Raises POP Levels in Blood

This finding presents us with a catch-22 situation. To get the toxins out of our bodies, we must lose weight to leach the toxins out of our body fat. But as soon as POPs enter our bloodstream during the leaching, they reach organs of our body, such as the brain and heart, potentially causing serious damage by triggering dementia or heart disease.

This research finding appeared in a 2013 study of 1,099 Americans who had their blood tested for the presence of seven POP compounds. The highest concentrations of the POPs were discovered in people who had lost the most weight over the previous decade, as opposed to people who had maintained their weight or gained weight during the same period. More extensive research is needed to determine the extent to which raised levels of circulating POPs directly cause health problems.[67]

Age-Specific Studies Linking Toxins and Obesity

Other medical studies have focused on toxin contamination and weight gain in specific age groups. For instance, in 2012 scientists measured the weight and levels of 21 POPs in 511 people who were 70 years old and re-measured weight and toxin levels again five years later. Abdominal obesity, defined as increased waist circumference, was found to be directly associated with concentrations of toxins, particularly PCBs, DDE, and dioxins.[68]

Another study of 90 young people in 2015, who were 18 to 30 years of age, measured levels of 32 POPs in blood over several decades. After 23 years of exposure to the accumulating POPs, all of the symptoms associated with metabolic syndrome, from weight gain to diabetes, intensified. The most health dangers, or toxin triggers, appeared between the ages of 48 and 55 years.[69]

OBESITY AND THE BRAIN

If asked, most people can list a number of effects on the body from being overweight. Most commonly you may hear that being overweight puts more pressure on the heart, and cholesterol levels may be higher in those carrying a few additional pounds. Some may ramble off some of the physical effects being overweight has on one's back or knees or maybe early fatigue from physical activity and weighing more than you are supposed to. While those are some of the common answers, do most people know that being overweight can actually cause problems with the brain?

Yes, being overweight can plague both mental health as well as the actual neural functions of the brain. An assistant professor of environmental and occupational health at Texas A&M, Ranjana Mehta, noted that atrophy and physical structure changes of the brain has been detected in overweight seniors. How about losing some of the brains memory capacity or failing to remember small details because of being overweight? This memory loss has been seen to play a double role when one forgets to literally watch what they eat or stay on a diet. These details can be glossed over easier research is showing. How about early, onset dementia? Lucy Cheke and her team from the University of Cambridge in England connected the dots between cardiovascular health from being overweight and a higher risk of Alzheimer's and early dementia. This is downright scary. If it isn't enough to know the downright dangers of being overweight and the game of life roulette overweight people are already playing, to lose a grasp on reality is in fact a chilling thought.

If this new research isn't sobering enough, there is also new research stating that being overweight can inhibit your sense of pleasure. This makes sense from a dietary point of view if we look at sugar. When the body consumes sugar, dopamine is released into the brain, which is a pleasure hormone. If your diet consists of an increased sugar intake, it only makes sense that the body would need more and more sugar to release more dopamine. This triggers the scary cycle of eating your way into happiness, especially when what you are eating is also causing you to gain weight.

This cycle often goes on in the body and the mind. Even when overweight persons know what they are doing is wrong, they continue the cycle, which often leads to depression, which leads back to eating for comfort and furthering the overweight epidemic. When we really think about it, of course, being overweight would cause problems in the brain. It is tremendously sad knowing that some of those afflicted with being overweight carry this additional emotional burden that comes with it. And with those emotional problems it seems that we are eating ourselves into depression and now facing mental problems much earlier in life. The burden of being overweight is hard enough without the mental baggage that goes along with it.

WE NEED A "TOXINS TO WEIGHT GAIN" AWARENESS

Even some of the more common ingredients added to our food supply by food manufacturers may be obesogens, acting as stimulators of fat tissue growth. One example is monosodium glutamate (MSG), often added to food to preserve its taste, particularly in Chinese restaurants, but also embedded in a wide variety of processed foods. Animal studies have found that MSG, when added to diets, results in quick fat growth, leading to obesity, alterations in liver function, accelerated inflammation, and symptoms associated with type 2 diabetes.[70]

We are continually exposed to natural toxins and synthetic chemical toxins every day—in the food we eat, air we breathe, water we drink, and items we touch. Learning more about how to identify these harmful impurities, and how to reduce our contact with them, is critical for making decisions to protect our future health.

Human exposure and reaction to natural toxins depends largely on how food is prepared. Cooking food breaks down many plant and animal (toxic) defenses. Also, the process of fermentation, in which microorganisms predigest a food to make it more edible, acts to disintegrate them.

The introduction of new foods and food preparation techniques throughout history has generated toxins and chemicals, many of which weren't discovered to be toxic until after generations of people had absorbed them. As an example, when heat is used to cook meat, the reaction can emit its own chemicals, such as char and nitrosamines. And, while heat may break down the toxic defenses present in the food being cooked, the chemicals produced can have a carcinogenic toxic effect on the body.

Toxins are even produced within the human body from simply living day to day, sometimes produced to battle foreign bacteria and viruses. These natural toxins can cause harm as they work to protect the body. But after their job is done, they are ultimately purified through biochemical processes.

All of these toxins are usually eliminated by the body without much adverse effect, but in the industrial age, pollution and food processing have increased the body's toxic burden considerably. The buildup of these toxins in the body is wreaking havoc on our health. As we know, humans have added thousands of new chemicals that pollute the air and water and can often end up concentrated in foods. Beyond this, food is laden with chemicals in the form of pesticides, processing agents, hormones, antibiotics, and other artificial ingredients.

According to an estimate from Mark Hyman, M.D., in his book *The Ultra Mind Solution,* "The average person consumes one gallon of neurotoxic pesticides and herbicides each year by eating conventionally grown fruits and vegetables." Imagine that! One gallon of pesticides and herbicides absorbed. The argument by chemical manufacturers, that tiny amounts of exposure to these toxins are harmless, begins to break down when you consider the toxic buildup in body fat that occurs over time from constant exposure to conventionally grown fruits and vegetables. The more body fat we accumulate over time; the more cell containers we carry around for toxins to congregate in.

By consuming any amount of conventionally grown fruits and vegetables, without taking toxins into account, humans are at risk of harming their bodies. Since pesticides are neurotoxic, and work by attacking insects' nervous systems, it is believed that ingesting large quantities of toxic pesticides from our food and environment may result in severe damage to our nerve processes.

Additionally, the continual flow of pollutants into water sources increases our risk of exposure to toxins. There are now hundreds of chemicals in municipal drinking water, including Prozac, Lipitor, and many other pharmaceutical and prescription drugs that may have adverse effects on the body and its functions, such as altering metabolism, which as we know causes weight gain.

As the body is endlessly exposed, these toxins can overwhelm the body's natural detoxification defenses. A slow accumulation of toxicity in the body over time may eventually undermine us both mentally and physically. Also keep in mind that most of the foods available today are not designed to support the body nutritionally, and the ubiquitous oversized portions poured onto our plates, lauded with "synthetic chemical additives, only add to the toxic burden and our weight gain.

OVERWEIGHT CHILDREN AT GREATEST RISK

Needless to say, children are the future of our species. The World Health Organization reported that overweight children are much more likely to become obese when they reach adulthood, and they are also much more likely than other children to suffer from cardiovascular diseases or diabetes at younger ages. The result is a greater likelihood of disability or premature death.

The fact that this health crisis has turned so viciously on our youth should be all the information required for us to take a stand. Being overweight, or excessively overweight, does prey on men, women, and children equally.

Excessive overweight is linked as a serious factor in more than 30 conditions that affect women, and these effects can show up at any stage of life. Many conditions, such as arthritis, deep vein thrombosis, obstetric and gynecological complications, and some cancers, have been identified as weight-related. Excessive weight in women has become the second largest cause of preventable death in the United States, following only tobacco-related illnesses. Breast cancer may be linked to weight issues in some women. At a minimum, being overweight creates greater susceptibility for breast cancer, according to research conducted over 16 years by The Nurses' Health Study, involving 95,256 nurses between 30 and 55 years of age. Weight gain after 18 years of age was associated with breast cancer incidence after menopause.

We need to remain aware that the rules of health have changed. The additional fat we carry around is a problem, but so are the hidden toxins stored in that fat.

HOW DO YOU MEASURE UP?

The term overweight actually refers to an individual weighing 10 percent or more of what is considered his or her recommended healthy weight, which is calculated by body mass index. This is often determined by large-scale population surveys. Obesity is a medical condition, a term used by both the medical establishment and the US government. According to the World Health Organization, the definition of obesity is: a medical condition in which excess fat has accumulated to the extent that it may have an adverse effect on health, leading to reduced life expectancy and/or increased health problems.

Are you overweight or obese? Although it is far from perfect, there is a tool used and developed by the government called the BMI chart. BMI stands for Body Mass Index. Remember, this is not something that was designed as a scare tactic. For some, it might even be a motivator. This chart is a general mathematical equation developed by the government to determine which category a person falls in, ranging from underweight to excessively overweight. The BMI is a simple equation using both height and weight to determine where one fits into a number of different weight categories. It will give most people a general feel for where they rank, according to government standards. It does not factor in several important facets such as muscle mass or other issues that may play a role in the outcome. To see where you are on the BMI chart, there are plenty of sites online that offer BMI calculators. The National Institutes of Health offers a BMI calculator anyone can access.[71]

See Calculate Your BMI–Standard BMI Calculator at: www.nhlbi.nih.gov/. . .wt/BMI/bmicalc.htm

There are four numeric categories used in the BMI chart. The chart's general range is from 18.5 to 30. If your number comes up at or below 18.5, you are considered underweight. If you find yourself between 18.5 and 24.9, you are within the normal, "healthy weight" category. From 25 to 29.9, you are considered overweight. Any number over 30 puts you in the obese group. BMIs calculated from 35 to 40 are considered severe obesity.

From 40 to 44.9, people find themselves in the category of morbid obesity, and anything above 50 is classified as super obesity. Generally speaking, super obesity usually means that a person is 100 or more pounds overweight. The government needed a way to generalize our ever-increasing waistlines. This is the current standard for determining a person's weight.

If you calculate your BMI and are in the healthy weight category, congratulations are in order. Maybe!

A healthy weight is a great first step but consider something you don't hear every day: being thin doesn't mean you're not fat. Talk about an oxymoron. Even if you are within the healthy weight guidelines, you could still have toxicity or be nutritionally deficient, and stressed out. There may even be hidden fat that doesn't show on the outside, called visceral fat. It's what's on the inside that counts.

Your Risk from Invisible Fat

It is believed that fat, undetectable by the naked eye, could pose huge health risks for those who think they are out of harm's reach. There are thin layers of visceral fat that surround our vital organs, such as the liver, pancreas, and heart called visceral fat. This type of fat is more dangerous than the outer fat visible on most overweight people.

In an *Associated Press* article from 2007, "Thin People May Be Fat Inside," Maria Cheng shared the dangers of judging health only by weight and general appearance. People can be dangerously misled about the quality of their health by critiquing only their appearance in the mirror. The article included the work of Dr. Jimmy Bell, a professor of molecular imaging in London. Since 1994 he has been creating "fat maps." Using MRI technology, Bell has scanned close to 800 people to determine where fat is stored in the body. A sleek outer appearance can be a giant misreading of a person's actual health. Dr. Bell concluded, "The whole concept of being fat needs to be redefined."

Bell contends that some people who are fat on the inside but seemingly thin on the outside could actually find themselves in a category closer to being excessively overweight from a health risk point of view. Often taking for granted their slim physiques, people think they can get away with eating bad fats, sugars, and so on. Because they don't see the weight gain, they often chalk it up to good genetics or fast metabolisms. The fact is, regardless of what the mirror portrays, everyone needs to find their own balance using both nutrition and exercise.

TDOS SYNDROME'S INTERCONNECTIONS MAGNIFY PROBLEMS

As Dr. Nicholas Messina points out, people who are thin can still be affected by the TDOS Syndrome. They are still susceptible to toxicity, nutritional deficiency, and stress. These three co-factors can also lead to the accumulation of visceral fat around the organs. Visceral fat produces pro-inflammatory mediators, which have been linked to cardiovascular disease, diabetes, and certain cancers. The journal of Hepatology (11 April 2008) reports evidence that visceral fat is linked to non-alcoholic fatty liver disease and metabolic syndrome Most doctors tend to treat the complications from excess fat accumulation, including hypertension, dyslipidemia, type 2 diabetes, and cardiovascular disease, in isolation, rather than focusing on the root problem. It is becoming increasingly clear that the primary cause of many of these problems is the accumulation of excess body fat stored as visceral fat in the abdominal cavity and the liver.

The rules have changed. Now it seems that BMI results are more of a starting point of reference. Just because you find yourself in the normal weight category, you may still be fat internally. Could this potentially be worse than actually showing the weight? While it is a great idea to eat healthy and exercise frequently, there's more to the story. Given what we have learned so far about the interconnectivity and magnification of The TDOS Syndrome co-factors, we should know by now that exercise and what we think is healthy eating will no longer be sufficient.

It's not just about food, calories, and exercise. Right now, we have all four co-factors of the TDOS Syndrome working against us at once. Until we find a way to defend against them, along with the reactions created by the synergy of these problems working together, any approach using diet and exercise alone will be inadequate in our quest to live healthier longer.

Some diet plans may work for a short time, but in the long run there is no diet or exercise machine out there that can withstand the lasting effects of the TDOS Syndrome on the body. The TDOS Syndrome is one of the primary causes of gaining weight. The four co-factors of TDOS combine and magnify its effects through a process called *interconnectivity*. This combined force is the reason we are losing the battle of the bulge, resulting in weight gain. We continue to fight this epidemic with outdated tools. We keep on generating solutions based on old tactics that don't take into account the new interconnectivity information. TDOS is the primary reason why the old health conversation, centered on the ideas we thought worked, is no longer adequate, nor effective.

That is why we must engage in a new health conversation.

For years I focused on calorie reduction and exercise to help my patients who were overweight and, according to the government, obese. The results were disappointing. I am now convinced that becoming overweight and obese is a multi-factorial condition and that toxicity, nutritional deficiency, and stress must be addressed together with diet and exercise for a meaningful and lasting outcome.

—NICHOLAS MESSINA, MD

Simply stated, a lack of nutrients in the body allows toxicity to run rampant by depriving the body's natural detoxification system of the essential nutrients needed to operate and remove toxins from our bodies.

Toxic obesogens are created and cannot be removed, due to the inadequate nutrient level. As a consequence, the nutrient deficiencies in our food supply are causing malnutrition in overweight children. When you think of overweight people, "malnourished" probably doesn't spring to mind. The truth is that it's more likely than not. When there is a lack of just one nutrient, the entire body chemistry can be thrown off kilter. According to Dr. Messina, there are really two types of hunger in the body: True physical hunger is triggered by the body's need for nutrients; psychological hunger is triggered by the need for immediate gratification, which is often satisfied for a short time by processed foods with a certain blend of fat, sugar, and salt. This satisfies the immediate perceived need but leads to the phenomenon of craving. The more we crave, the more we eat these foods. The more we eat these types of foods, the less we satisfy physiologic hunger and the more we eat.

Most people seek out the food that will serve them best at any given time. Every day, we work to make life easier and more efficient.

In the body, we cut corners with sugar and caffeine to get us going. In reality, we are satisfying the wrong hunger in the body and selling ourselves short. A body supplied with proper nutrition, versus one fueled by stimulants like sugar and caffeine, will not end up in the same category of health.

We are conditioned to grab that pre-packaged, processed-to-the-tenth-degree granola bar or chug a 16-ounce energy drink with triple caffeine and an ingredient list scripted in what reads like a foreign language. There is a simple saying, "If you can't pronounce an ingredient, you should probably not eat it." Another ingredient list guideline: The shorter, the better.

DIETS CAN PRODUCE WEIGHT GAIN?

Low-calorie diets increase stress on the body, because by lowering the calories, you are probably also drastically decreasing the nutritional density of the calories you do consume. The body becomes stressed out trying to allocate these nutritionally bankrupt calories to meet all of its needs. The body reacts to stress by increasing cortisol, so cutting calories actually increases cortisol levels. I know that sounds counter-intuitive on some level, but it is our biological reality.

When you start a diet, often one of the first steps is to lower caloric intake. We know that when calories are reduced, nutritional deficiency comes into play because generally the foods we eat are sadly lacking in nutrient density. So in addition to nutritional deficiency, dieting adds to the stress on the body thus stimulating cortisol levels.

According to the *Gale Encyclopedia of Medicine*, cortisol is a hormone released by the cortex (outer portion) of the adrenal gland when a person is under stress. What we are learning is that when cortisol is chronic and unrelenting, it can cause the body to store fat and decrease lean muscle development, which over time can also serve to increase weight gain. Cortisol is the hormone that's released based on stress in the body. Yes, there are times when it plays an important role. When stress and cortisol become chronic, however, it can be extremely dangerous to our health. We now know that cortisol is a contributing factor to weight gain.

Chronic cortisol causes the body to retain fat and gain weight. As the body begins to produce cortisol, it also stops burning fat. At the same time, the body slows the secretion of the key anabolic hormones—DHEA, testosterone, and the growth hormone—that help the body burn fat for fuel.

Why Low-Calorie Diets Cause Stress

Following a low-calorie diet places stress on the body, ultimately leading to rebound weight gain after the diet is stopped and is completely opposite of the desired outcome. Cutting calories was once the fail-safe way to melt extra pounds. Not anymore. When the body is stressed, it burns fewer calories. In some people, it may even cause an increased appetite, especially for carbohydrates, which can increase stress levels thus increasing cortisol and further fat storage. It's a tragic and scary downward spiral that most of us are not even aware is happening.

It should be clear now that dieting and cutting calories (while at the same time ignoring the nutritional deficit created) is a waste of time and can lead to an increase in stress, potentially making you more likely to gain weight. Calories are not necessarily what you think. A calorie is really just a unit of energy. One calorie is the amount of heat required to raise the temperature of one kilogram of water by one degree Celsius. In the US the popular use of the term calorie actually means the kilocalorie, sometimes called the kilogram calorie. The large calorie (equal to 1,000 calories) is used in measuring the calorific heating or metabolizing value of foods. Thus, the "calories" counted for dietary reasons are in fact kilocalories.

The amount of calories indicated for a given food expresses how much energy is supplied to the body in consuming it. Most health professionals and the general public associate calories with whatever they drink or eat. As we know, calories cannot be directly equated to levels of nutrition. We put so much attention on calories in food, yet the body does not count calories. It responds to nutrients.

Calories can only be measured in a formal laboratory setting. The human body has no idea how to calculate the importance of one calorie. Instead, the body's role is to dissect the nutritional value of a calorie. This becomes apparent when you compare 1,000 calories of fruits and vegetables to 1,000 calories of processed foods like potato chips and candy bars. Clearly, each diet consists of the same amount of calories from a basic measuring standpoint. However, each choice would result in two very different outcomes for the body. The body can only use the nutrition that's available to function as efficiently as possible.

A study compared three different eating patterns: a low-fat diet, a low-glycemic-index diet, and a low-carbohydrate diet. The findings illustrated that all calories are not alike from a metabolic perspective. When any major nutrient was avoided or restricted, there was a metabolic consequence noted. It was suggested to focus not on the quantity of calories but rather on the quality of nutrients in the calories.

—NICHOLAS MESSINA, MD

Journal of the American Medical Association, 6.27.12

WHAT THOSE EXCESS POUNDS COST US

Humans are faced with a two-headed monster when it comes to being overweight. First, it affects our overall health and well-being. Second, excessive weight gain carries a substantial economic impact, and even moderate weight gain affects the bottom line. We simply cannot afford to pay for all this excess weight.

Research estimates that people who are moderately overweight will increase health care costs by 20 percent to 30 percent compared to those at an ideal weight. Medical treatments for overweight individuals, along with conditions and related health problems will cost this country billions of dollars a year. By one estimate, the US spent $190 billion in health care expenses in 2005 on the excessively overweight and their associated conditions. This number doubled previous estimates. The enormity of this economic burden and the huge toll that excess weight takes on health and well-being are raising global awareness that more must be done to stem the rising tide of this colossal problem.

An analysis prepared by Scott Kahan, director of the National Center for Weight & Wellness at George Washington University, pegged the total cost of obesity—including direct medical and non-medical services, decreased worker productivity, disability, and premature death—at $305.1 billion annually.[72]

What makes this research on excessively overweight people so alarming? All signs indicate that people are really starting to let themselves go. Each day, people seem to care less about being fat. This attitude will only spike the amount of money spent on health care in America. If the current trends are not altered, it is estimated that in 2018, Americans will shell out $344 billion on health-care costs attributable to our weight problems. That's not even the total amount spent on health care, just the portion attributable to how we have overfed ourselves.

There are so many startling facts emerging in this new wave of overweight that it's hard to stay informed of them all. Every day, new research lands on the front page of our newspapers, magazines, and websites. It is estimated that for the first time ever there are more people who are excessively overweight than just a few pounds over the limit. The number of excessively overweight people has increased almost 12 percent from where it was in 1994 and has officially surpassed those who have had to notch one new hole in their belts.

There is no solution to the weight-gain dilemma until we understand the entire situation. Once you realize the long-term effects of being overweight, you can begin to address what really causes it. Excess weight increases the risk of developing conditions such as diabetes, heart disease, osteoarthritis, and certain cancers. It will reduce your lifespan. Those who are unable to control their weight may be headed into a state of obesity. In June 2013 the medical community officially classified obesity as a disease.

EXCESS WEIGHT: A GATEWAY TO DISEASE

As scary as cancer may be, it is also chilling to learn that women dealing with weight problems are at risk of harming their babies' health. Not only have birth defects in children been associated with excessively overweight women but also infertility rates have been increasing. Once again, the decisions currently being made based on weight and health play a critical role in future generations.

Cardiovascular disease is another major health problem associated with overweight women. Excessive weight is a determinant for all risk factors associated with heart disease. Not long ago, cardiovascular disease was categorized as more of a man's disease. It has been determined that overweight females are positively linked with cardiovascular disease and its risk factors in middle and older-age groups. This does not excuse males from the discussion. Men with excessive visceral fat will see a substantial increase in the risk of conditions like heart disease and diabetes.

DON'T FORGET STRESS ALSO MAKES US FAT

Pent-up stress leads to cortisol remaining in the body, resulting in chronic levels of cortisol that trigger the body to increase insulin production. Simply by doing its job, an elevated insulin level causes the body to store fat. As I emphasize throughout this book, being overweight is not simply about overeating and under-exercising. The by-products of stress, explained in detail in the next chapter, also contribute to weight gain.

Chronic cortisol, a by-product of stress, the "S" in The TDOS Syndrome, will raise insulin levels, helping the body store fat and leading to weight gain. Dr. Nicholas Messina makes the point that we have been looking through the wrong end of the telescope. We have focused on treating overweight and obesity as if these conditions were from a single cause, without taking into account the contributing factors of toxicity, nutritional deficiency, and stress.

Our obesity epidemic speaks volumes about the need to change our health strategies. In 2013 *The American Journal of Clinical Nutrition* published some startling statistics revealing that US adults have been eating steadily fewer calories for almost a decade. Despite this reduction in calorie intake, the population's rate of weight gain continues to increase. The researchers were stumped by these results—but you should not be, after reading this book. Our health focus needs to be on toxins, nutritional deficiency, and stress, if we are to bring the ravenous weight-gain monster under control.

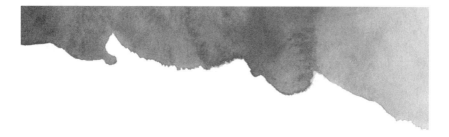

PART FOUR

Co-Factor S—**Stress**

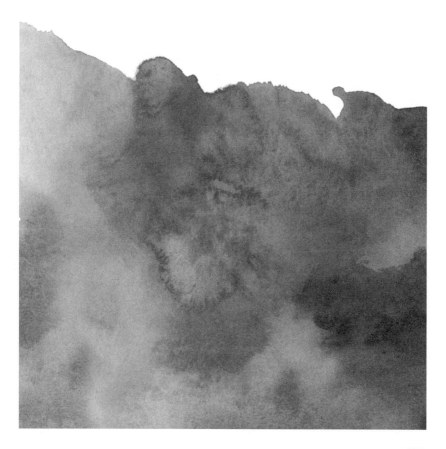

Co-Factor S—Stress

Chronic Stress Respects
No One's Boundaries

Over a lifetime, chronic stress can build up like toxic barnacles on sea rock, exacting a silent and deadly toll on the mind and body. My experience in this regard may, unfortunately, ring true for many of you. Stress nearly killed me, before I became aware of it as a TDOS co-factor. What I discovered through my research was that I had paid a high price during my life because I never realized that feelings of fear, anxiety, depression, and insecurity were just names and disguises for chronic stress. How I nearly wound up on death's doorstep in 2003, which I described earlier in this book, has a backstory.

As a child, I was given last rites four times before the age of six. This was due to high fevers that sent me into convulsions until I would stop breathing. Those alarming experiences triggered a life-long feeling of stress about being around doctors and hospitals. At the age of 11, my parents divorced, and I ended up with my mother when I wanted to be with my father. During the emotionally stress-ful and bitter custody battle, I ran away from my mother in Nevada and escaped to my father's side in Michigan, creating a rift with my mother that took years to heal.

As a member of the highly competitive University of Colorado ski team, alongside Olympic medal winners Billy Kidd and Jimmy Heuga, I developed a fear of success, which instilled its own unique brand of stress. Even after an injury ended my ski racing career, this fear of success became an undercurrent of stress that continued to plague me in all my professional endeavors.

In adulthood, I grew a custom cabinetry business into a large and thriving enterprise, but only by working with full focus and dedication seven days a week. Every weekend was miserable; by Sunday I was a nervous wreck since I knew and dreaded what was in store for me on Monday. There was no such thing as a day off, or being sick. I had to do what was required to keep the business growing, day after day, week after week, month after month. It became so bad that every night, almost without fail, I would buy a half gallon of inexpensive red wine and drink most of it. And like clockwork, I would wake up in a cold sweat at two or three o'clock in the morning and toss and turn until 5:00 a.m. when it was time to get up.

The pressure, the stress, and the anxiety were literally sapping the life force out of me. Yet I had no clue because I had accepted it as normal. I just knew that to keep up with my workload, to generate the income needed to support the family and lifestyle I wanted, I had to toil 80 to 90 hours a week without fail. Many entrepreneurs and all of you workaholics and stressaholics reading these words can probably relate to what I am saying. Chronic stress can literally consume your life, and you begin to think of it as merely a price that must be paid for achieving—and maintaining—that success.

Without the terrible, eye-opening news about my state of health given to me by my doctor in 2003, I am not sure that I would have survived. That was my wake-up call. I had to make major changes. There was no other option. There is an old saying "When the pain to remain the same is greater than the pain to change, then we change."

All too often it's a life crisis, in the form of a health decline that becomes the necessary motivation for us to relinquish toxic lifestyle habits. I am clear that without this stress-related breakdown in my case, I would not be writing this book and sharing the message of what I discovered.

Chronic stress is a hell of a lot more than just a periodic knot in your stomach. It wears many faces. It descends on us disguised as anxiety, depression, fatigue, loss of motivation, and insecurity, and it evolves over time to become a major factor in the onset of many disease processes and the acceleration of aging.

The crazy part about stress is that we need a certain minimum amount of it, and the hormone cortisol that it produces, to stay functionally activated in setting and achieving goals. It's just that there is a tipping point, one so delicate that most of us don't know the warning signs to indicate when the tip-over has been initiated.

What no one needs, and what our bodies cannot long tolerate, is unrelenting chronic stress at the levels that nearly killed me. Added to the other co-factors of the TDOS Syndrome, chronic stress acts like a seismic disturbance, further cracking apart our foundation of health stability. Let's take a closer look at how this interaction between stress and the co-factors occurs.

STRESS IS A VICIOUS CYCLE

As the fourth co-factor of the TDOS Syndrome, stress is a vicious and, for the most part, often-ignored killer, *perhaps* because it plays so many varied and complex roles in human biochemistry. Stress in our lives is much more complicated than it appears on the surface. It's not just the aggravation of rush-hour traffic, nor having too much to do and too little time to do it.

When stress becomes chronic, it's a silent killer all by itself. It's also one outcome of the increasing level of toxicity and nutrient deficiency in the human body. Taken together, this alteration in the body's biochemistry leads to weight gain. Then too much weight adds stress to the body, causing the release of hormones that prevent the body from losing weight. We find ourselves in an endless downward spiral that continues to get worse. The body requires specific nutrients to offset stress and, because we face a massive nutritional deficiency, those nutrients are not available to us and our stress worsens. It plays havoc with hormones, especially the stress hormone, cortisol. It is a complex and endless loop.

The magnitude of this problem and the negative health effects are much larger than any one of the co-factors alone might lead us to believe. Each co-factor in TDOS magnifies the deleterious effects of each of the others on our health. Traditional approaches in health care tackle problems individually and defensively. That is short-sighted and usually ineffective, when it involves treating the manifestations of the TDOS Syndrome.

EVERY THOUGHT CAN BE A POTENTIAL "LION"

Let's start with a tidy definition of stress from Shawn M. Talbott, PhD, from his book *The Cortisol Connection: Why Stress Makes You Fat and Ruins Your Health–And What You Can Do About It.* This is one of the best books I've read on stress, specifically on the many-faceted roles cortisol plays in stress's negative effects on our health. Talbott defines stress as "what you feel when life's demands outweigh your ability to meet those demands."

The original explanation of stress is the "fight or flight" response, such as when an antelope runs from a lion. The "flight" reaction is powered by stress. Assuming the antelope does not become the lion's lunch, it goes into recovery mode after its "flight." The stress response in humans works much the same way. That "fight or flight" solution may work on the Savannah, but not for us. Today, there's no recovery time from endless stressful situations. Every thought or relationship is a potential lion.

Stress is a natural process in the body that is needed for the body to function properly. As stated earlier, the body naturally produces a hormone called cortisol whose job is to manage the body's systems when it encounters stress. Although stress is part of our human functionality, our bodies are not designed for constant reaction to stress, especially when it haunts us day and night, 24 hours a day, seven days a week, every day of the year. Over time, the response to such unrelenting stress does real damage to every cell in the human body.

"Some stress is good," observed a 2011 commentary in the journal *Environmental Health Perspectives*. "Human systems are designed with an autonomic nervous system that responds to stress by stimulating the release of the hormones adrenaline (to speed heart rate, pump up blood pressure, and mobilize energy) and cortisol (to replenish energy supplies and prime the immune system to combat threats.) This type of stress has been called 'positive stress.'"[73]

But if the "fight or flight" response brought on by stress "continues for too long, a constant flow of the hormones may 'reset' the immune system so that it either stays revved up or becomes suppressed," the commentary continued. There are differences between acute and chronic stress to keep in mind. Acute stress may last for hours or days, whereas chronic stress lasts for weeks or years. It is primarily this chronic stress that seems to interact with toxic chemicals and pollutants to magnify health risks for people who are exposed, particularly by warping the immune system and its response to body invaders.

> . . . the original purpose of stress was to save our lives. When a caveman or cave woman was being chased by a lion, tiger, or bear, the stress response would kick in, providing the energy necessary to allow the cave person to run or fight. The problem is that in modern day instead of having real stressors, we have mostly imagined stressors, that is, dangers that our mind conjures up or which pose no true threat to our survival. The problem is that the body cannot differentiate between what is imagined and what is real. The same brain centers light up whether the danger is real or imagined. Therefore, we react to whatever we view in our imagination.
>
> **—ROBERT L. FRIEDMAN, MA**
> **Clinical Director of Stress Solutions, Inc.**

OUR STRESS EPIDEMIC

Perpetual or chronic stress is a serious obstacle to maintaining good health. The human body and its internal systems, including the nervous system and the endocrine system (our hormones), aren't set up to cope with the unique set of stressful challenges to everyday life in the twenty-first century. Health and medical research data collected during the past 20 to 30 years continues to affirm this.

Robert Friedman, Clinical Director of Stress Solutions, Inc., identifies four categories of sources for stress: "environmental stressors, social stressors, physiological stressors, and our thinking process." Environmental stressors include drastic temperature changes, loud noise levels, toxic chemical odors, and even mosquitoes. Sources of stress in the social sphere tend to involve relations between loved ones, friends, and co-workers. Housing, finances, public speaking, and school are other examples. The physical body is the site for physiological stressors and that can be evidenced in back pain, migraines, or cancer. "The final factor, which often creates more stress than the last three, is your thoughts. We have learned it is the *perception* of an event which creates the most stress, even more so than the actual event," writes Friedman. So your thoughts alone can stress you out. (No lions required.)

Money and work are regularly ranked at the top of the list of stressors for most people. These socio-economic factors play a huge role in the unrelenting levels of societal stress. The American Psychological Association has been surveying the American population about stress every year since 2007. The APA's 2012 report states, "Top sources of stress include money (69 percent), work (65 percent), the economy (61 percent), family responsibilities (57 percent), relationships (56 percent), family health problems (52 percent) and personal health concerns (51 percent)."[74]

BY THE NUMBERS: THE COSTS OF STRESS

Stress is expensive! The CDC estimates that 80 percent of all health-care dollars are spent on stress-related issues, and the American Medical Association estimates that stress is a factor in 80 to 85 percent of all health problems. As Dr. Talbott tells us in *The Cortisol Connection*, American businesses lose about $200 billion to $300 billion each year due to productivity losses from stress-related issues.

Some of the most common stress-related health problems include stomach problems like ulcers, high blood pressure, heart disease, asthma, allergies, cancer, and even headaches. One of the reasons stress is so expensive, according to the Centers for Disease Control, is the fact that our immune systems are suppressed when we're under constant, chronic stress. As a result, the body is more susceptible to diseases like the common cold and flu.

Stress is also the reason for many of the medications consumed, both prescription and over-the-counter drugs. Some estimate that as many as 95 million Americans take medication for some disease related to stress or with its roots in this epidemic. The American Institute of Stress in Yonkers, New York, estimates that 90 percent of all visits to doctors are for stress-related disorders.[75]

CONSTANT STRESS = CONSTANT CORTISOL

These stressors of daily life all take a toll—real situations, problems, worries, and anxieties. As we fret over worst-case scenarios, infinite rewind loops play in our mind. Such chronic, unrelenting stress elevates cortisol, the stress hormone. Negative consequences play out when levels of cortisol rise unabated.

The body's biochemistry is a complex list of multiple interconnections, as we have seen throughout our consideration of the TDOS Syndrome. One of the body's most complex interrelationships around weight gain and stress revolves around cortisol. Cortisol levels affect the breakdown of glucose, protein, and fat and have anti-inflammatory and anti-allergy effects, according to the National Institutes of Health. It helps the body maintain physiological functioning, especially when in a state of trauma. Without it, the body would not be able to deal with stress.[76]

The problem with humans in our "always-on" state is that our fearful and stressful thoughts never entirely subside. Our bodies deal with the stress of bills to pay or fear of losing a job as if a lion was relentlessly on the chase. Our human bodies have "adapted" to deal with apparent psychological or mental threats in the same way that an antelope deals with physical threats. So the switch for cortisol streaming into our system is rarely if ever turned off. The result is that it wreaks havoc with our health.

For the sake of your health, I urge you to take cortisol seriously and understand how it plays a role in the retention of fat cells. Chronic stress and chronic cortisol cause ripple effects on your health, causing an invisible tsunami of deterioration inside your body.

STRESS AND OVERWEIGHT CO-FACTORS MAGNIFY

If you were being chased by a lion, your cortisol would turn off fat-burning and digestion. It amplifies processes to give your body immediate energy from sources like glucose, simple sugars that give your body the energy to run away from the lion. But when cortisol tries to deal with your chronic stress of everyday "always-on" life, guess what? The message the body keeps receiving is *not* to burn fat. This chronic stress and chronically elevated cortisol are crucial factors in our inability to lose fat. They contribute to the epidemic of being overweight.

As we examine each of the four parts of the TDOS, we observe that the interactions among the three other co-factors all conspire to magnify the destructive capabilities of chronic stress and chronic cortisol. There are several other effects on the human body from chronic cortisol that should be noted.

Chronic cortisol draws amino acids from skeletal muscles, as a way to generate that "quick energy" the body needs in an emergency. This causes muscle loss. It's basically as if our bodies "eat" our muscles. With a lowered muscle mass, courtesy of chronic cortisol, it becomes even harder to lose weight because the body, even at rest, burns more calories to sustain muscles than to maintain fat. So chronic cortisol leads to fewer calories being burned, while telling the body to hang onto fat, and even collect more of it!

Chronic cortisol release is also one of the culprits leading to lower bone density, in addition to numerous other chronic health issues and health problems without identifiable causes. Are you aware of diseases with no known causes? These are basically medical mysteries—things like chronic fatigue syndrome, fibromyalgia, and IBS (irritable bowel syndrome). When your doctor isn't sure why you're sick, she might describe your illness as "idiopathic," doctor-speak for "of unknown causes."

ELEVATED CORTISOL, HSD, AND ABDOMINAL FAT

The Cortisol Connection offers clear explanations, backed by research, about these complex biochemical interconnections. Dr. Talbott, an expert on nutritional biochemistry, has taught me a tremendous amount about stress, chronic stress, and its by-products that are killing us: chronic elevated levels of cortisol and high levels of HSD (short for 11-betas-hydroxysteroid-dehydrogenase-1). HSD is an enzyme active in metabolic processes. HSD levels practically demand that the body retain fat, along with elevated insulin.

Chronic elevated cortisol plus HSD leads to a whole host of problems. Together, they are a major contributor to being overweight and the health problems that arise from being overweight. Again, here's a situation where the co-factors contribute and magnify the ill effects of each other in our deteriorating health.

HSD amplifies the negative effects of continual high amounts of cortisol circulating in our body. Research demonstrates that not only are high levels of cortisol detrimental to health but also cortisol can be at an acceptable level in the body's general system and still appear in certain cells in high amounts. While HSD is in nearly all cells, researchers show a correlation between cell-level elevated cortisol and the location of high and active amounts of HSD, especially within abdominal fat cells.

Together, cortisol plus HSD make weight loss even more difficult, while increasing the risk for diabetes, high blood pressure, and elevated levels of cholesterol. As Talbott notes in *The Cortisol Connection*, "As you struggle to lose weight, your fat cells increase their HSD activity, leading to more cortisol, a stronger signal to store fat and a gradual return to your pre-diet body weight."

EAT LESS, WEIGH MORE

Dieting, or even thinking about dieting, increases stress. Stress brings on cortisol and cortisol tells the body not to burn fat but to store it. It's a key factor to gaining weight, especially in the abdominal area. Not all fat is created equal. Fat carried in the abdominal area increases the risks for other health problems.

Talbott cites studies that reveal that stress and cortisol increase in the body when people go on low-calorie diets. Researchers from the University of Birmingham, in England, studied people following diets consisting of 800 calories a day over the course of ten or more weeks saw major metabolic effects on the body. This strategy of low-calorie dieting significantly increased cortisol levels throughout the body and also increased HSD activity within fat cells by 3.4 times.

Similarly, the Division of Cardiovascular Medicine at the University of Arkansas connects HSD and stress response to being overweight. In essence, the more you try to diet, the more stress you feel, and the more cortisol goes into your system, essentially turning off the body's ability to burn fat.

The National Institutes of Health (NIH), one of the world's top medical research centers, also studied HSD and obesity. The institute found that HSD activity was higher in obese people. NIH research has given credence to what others have observed—that people can gain weight even when it does not seem to correlate to the amount of food they consume.

Again, the by-product of a chronic high level of cortisol is that HSD escalates in response to this. HSD ratchets up our ability to tolerate these high levels of cortisol. At the same time, too much cortisol causes systemic health problems. We see yet another example of the magnification of co-factors of TDOS working in concert with horrible effects.

In some studies, people with high stress and lots of abdominal stress fat had normal or low levels of cortisol in their blood (or urine or saliva), indicating that there was no systemic cortisol overexposure. What we now know is that certain enzymes are deregulated in obesity—most notably the HSD enzymes in fat tissue—effectively leading to a "high" cortisol level within fat cells at all times.

—DR. SHAWN TALBOTT
The Cortisol Connection

STRESS, EATING, AND INSULIN

Cortisol's original function is to get the body to replenish its nutritional reserves after a stressful event. With both stress and cortisol at chronically high levels, it's like a hunger that never disappears. The body does not feel sated when we feed it, and we always want more. In part, this stems from the nutritional deficiency in our food.

Whether the body reacts based on the original intent of this stress-cortisol system, or from the habits we've developed or, most likely, a combination of both, one of the common human responses to stress is to eat, especially those carb-laden "comfort foods." Unfortunately, those are exactly the foods that, if eaten regularly and over an extended period, can cause insulin levels to get off-kilter. An overabundance of insulin, also a hormone, can wreak havoc with cellular health.

Insulin is best known for its role in managing blood sugar in the body's cells. Diabetes results when the system doesn't function properly and leaves excess sugar in the blood. According to Talbott, when cells resist insulin, the body, in turn, needs extra insulin in order to move sugar into the cells to create energy.

INSULIN CAN TEAM UP WITH CORTISOL
TO STORE FAT

Talbott also identifies the important role that insulin plays in storing nutrients for future use. In this way, insulin partners with cortisol within our stressful lives and can have a negative impact. Together, they amplify the signals to our bodies to store more fat and don't burn what has already accumulated. And so around and around we go.

This hard-working insulin hormone can then cause cells to stop responding. When cells stop responding, it can become dangerous. The body gets confused and starts to "eat" the muscle cells instead of burning fats. This is the slippery slope to type 2 diabetes.

HOW YOUR METABOLISM IS AFFECTED

Stress and hormones have a profound effect on your metabolism, or how your body obtains fuel. We've seen how stress ultimately causes the body to store and hang onto excess fat, with the hormones cortisol and insulin working in tandem.

In the catabolic state, your body breaks down tissue for energy while storing fat. (Among the by-products of this process is oxidation.) The culprit in this breakdown—or catabolic state—is cortisol, sometimes referred to as a catabolic hormone. While many hormones tend to decrease as we age, cortisol seems to increase.

In the anabolic metabolism state, your body builds or repairs tissue by burning fats. Dr. Talbott further examines these hormonal interconnections at great length, explaining how stress makes people gain weight through "excessive secretion" of cortisol "*a reduced secretion of key anabolic hormones* such as DHEA, testosterone and growth hormone."

Catabolic metabolism is also triggered by nutritional deficiency. The body is not just looking for calories to be satisfied. It is much more important to prevent catabolic metabolism by ensuring you intake the minimum number of nutrients. We saw in the chapter on deficiency that getting enough nutrients from food is almost impossible. And, not only can nutritional deficiency lead to catabolic metabolism but also it leads to weight gain and obesity. The interconnections are mind-boggling.

The entire process of cannibalizing our muscle and tendon tissues for that "quick fix" for glucose (simple sugars) to activate our "fight or flight" stress response, while storing extra fat and not burning fat, turns out to look a lot like how the body reacts when it's put on an all-protein diet. Experts say that in order for the brain to function properly, it needs four grams of sugar from carbohydrates converted into glucose every four hours. The brain is predominately fueled by glucose. Energy for the brain comes only from water, salt, and glucose.

If the brain does not receive glucose from available carbohydrates, it creates a catabolic metabolism. It draws from your lean muscle cells for fuel by converting those cells into glucose by a process called gluconeogenesis. This is how catabolic metabolism occurs.

To make matters worse, the lack of nutrients in our foods create more stress for our bodies. Cortisol levels rise and fat-burning gets blocked, all contributing to additional triggering of catabolic metabolism. Experts repeatedly say that an all-protein diet, even if it promotes weight loss, can stimulate a cascade of negative health side effects.

CONNECTING THE DOTS

Unchecked dangerous levels of cortisol has many negative effects on the body. Ignoring it has devastating consequences—and not just on our waistlines. From the research it's clear that chronic and sustained high levels of the hormone cortisol lead to accelerated aging. Accelerated aging is the worst possible side effect of cortisol. According to Dr. Nicholas Perricone, "It is not surprising that we in the anti-aging field call cortisol 'the death hormone,' because it is truly associated with old age and disease."[77]

Chronic stress and chronic high amounts of cortisol work together, causing a multiplying effect in the body. A chronic high level of cortisol predisposes the body to fat storage and weight gain, which leads to the natural process of oxidative stress that is intensified in the whirlwind of TDOS.

Oxidative Stress

Oxidative stress is the total burden placed on our bodies by the constant production of free radicals in the normal course of metabolism plus whatever other pressures the environment brings to bear (natural and artificial radiation, toxins in air, food and water; and other sources of oxidizing activity, such as tobacco smoke).

Oxidative stress, although a normal function in the body, is also increasing its destruction partly due to the perfect storm of all these co-factors of TDOS coming together. Combined, these co-factors magnify the damage caused by oxidative stress in the human body. According to research from the National Institute of Health, over-weight and obesity can trigger oxidative stress. We also know that chronic stress and chronic cortisol are among the interconnected co-factors leading to this constant weight gain.[78]

According to the NIH, oxidative stress and chronic inflammation caused by obesity are the main components in the development of diabetes and insulin resistance. However, these factors aren't directly to blame for weight gain and the increase in tissue mass. Our nutri-tionally deficient food inhibits the body from producing enough of the antioxidant enzymes that "tame" or "clean" the free radicals. Antioxi-dants are able to give the free radical molecules the extra electron they are missing, thus destroying the ability for the free radicals to damage the healthy cells. Nutrients must be present in sufficient quantities for antioxidant enzymes to perform their job and reduce free radi-cals in the body. If there are not enough nutrients, these antioxidant enzymes cannot remove the free radicals. Anti-aging scientists believe that high amounts of free radicals are a major contributing factor to accelerating the aging process. That is an outcome none of us want, since it clearly will interfere with any plans to live healthier longer.

COMPLEX INTERCONNECTIONS

Stress is arguably the most complex of the TDOS Syndrome's destruc-tive co-factors. Its lethal biochemical interconnections at the cellular level combined with its interactions with the other co-factors are mind boggling. Stress is both a cause and effect that magnifies all the other co-factors.

First, stress leads to chronically elevated levels of cortisol, which some call the "death hormone." We eat more when stressed and gain even more weight. Together, these lead to the second by-product: high insulin levels. This can cause health problems such as diabetes and even plays a role in heart disease. Third, chronic stress and elevated cortisol are part of accelerated aging. That process is further sped up by increased levels of oxidative stress, "rusting from the inside out." And although antioxidants can mitigate the free radicals released by cellular level respiration, the nutritional deficiency of our food—now stripped of its trace minerals—hinders our bodies from providing enough antioxidants to deal with these cell-damaging free radicals. Damaged cells lead to a host of other conditions and diseases, even premature death. When we connect the dots, the undeniable scientific evidence clearly illustrates the powerful link between these co-factors that together negatively impact our wellness potential.

WHAT THE SCIENTIFIC EVIDENCE REVEALS

Stress and the other three TDOS co-factors of toxins, nutrient deficiencies, and overweight unite in some unexpected and disturbing ways, as you will see from the following research study findings. They create the processes that ultimately lead to weight gain, malnutrition, and disease.

Did you know that overweight and obese men (and probably women, too) secrete large levels of stress hormones after eating, making them more susceptible to cardiovascular disease and type 2 diabetes? In a 2013 study presented to the 95th meeting of The Endocrine Society, the scientific organization devoted to research on hormones, scientists from Australia described how they tested 19 normal weight men and 17 overweight or obese men, by having their salivary cortisol concentrations measured during, before, and after a meal. Compared to normal weight men, the overweight or obese volunteers saw their cortisol levels increase by 51 percent, indicating their adrenal glands were working overtime, as if in response to a stressful situation.

Further studies will need to determine if the same holds true for women, though there is no reason to believe there would be a significant difference in the sexes.

"This research indicates that when we are carrying excess fat stores, we may also be exposing our bodies to increased levels of the stress hormone cortisol every time we have a meal," observed a study coauthor, Anne Turner, PhD. "If overweight and obese individuals have an increase in cortisol every time they ingest food, they may be at greater risk of developing stress-related diseases, such as cardiovascular disease, type 2 diabetes, depression and anxiety."[79]

To illustrate the link between stress-related cortisol levels and cardiovascular disease, scientists writing in a 2013 issue of the *Journal of Clinical Endocrinology & Metabolism* revealed how they measured scalp hair cortisol in 283 elderly people (average age of 75), who lived in a retirement community, and compared those levels with their diagnosed histories of cardiovascular disease. There was a clear link between high cortisol, as measured in hair samples, and cardiovascular disease risk, which should not be surprising given previous research showing that many elderly populations experience high stress levels due to anxiety and loneliness.[80]

Nutrient deficiencies also play an interactive role with stress among elderly populations. For example, a 2015 study in the journal *Public Health Nutrition* sampled more than 1,500 men and women, aged 65-87 years, for zinc deficiencies and found more than 30 percent of those who were at risk for malnutrition had such a nutrient deficiency. Other studies have shown that malnutrition among senior citizens contributes to mental health problems. Nutrient deficiency in this already vulnerable population can only add to their total burden of oxidative stress, as has been previously explained.[81]

Studies targeting other age groups, particularly children and their mothers, have uncovered compelling evidence that stress and pollution, both in the form of chemicals and air particles, interact to increase body weight. In a 2016 study for the science journal *Stress*, a group of 70 women and their children living in a disadvantaged community exposed to high levels of pollutants had their stress levels and body mass indexes measured and compared. Perceived Stress Scale scores were positively associated with higher body mass, which in turn were positively linked to high hair cortisol levels.[82]

An even larger study from Australia in 2013 evaluated stress and obesity in 1,382 women (18 to 46 years of age) living in socioeconomically disadvantaged neighborhoods. "Higher perceived stress in women was associated with a higher body mass index and increased odds of being obese," the research team concluded.[83]

What do stressed-out people in polluted neighborhoods mostly eat? Nutritionally deficient junk and fast foods, of course. A *British Journal of Nutrition* study found that "stress drives salt intake ... chronic stress was associated with increased consumption of snack foods, which included highly salty snacks." In fact, over the past few decades, the level of stress in any society can be measured by its levels of salt intake and the resulting dramatic rise in high blood pressure statistics.[84]

Returning to pollution and stress as disease triggers, a series of scientific studies have examined the relationships between stress and toxins in the air, and the range of resulting health problems. Take the incidence of asthma, for instance. A huge study in the *Proceedings of the National Academy of Sciences* examined 2,497 children, aged five to nine years, with no history of asthma when the study began. After three years of follow-up, it was found that "children from stressful households are more susceptible to the effects of traffic-related pollution," and that exposure to the stress and air toxins "significantly" affects the development of asthma.[85]

Chronic psychological stress "might enhance a child's vulnerability to certain chemical exposures," wrote the authors of a 2011 study in the journal *Environmental Health Perspectives*, "contributing to effects that later show up as asthma, neurodevelopmental disorders, cardiovascular diseases, obesity, cancer, and other problems."[86] Commenting on this study, Deborah Cory-Slechta, a professor of environmental medicine at the University of Rochester School of Medicine, noted: "We know some chemicals interact with stress, but we really don't know how broadly such interactions may occur across chemicals."

There are still many unknowns and medical science has a lot more work to do in drawing the TDOS connections tighter and, most especially, in understanding how and why the synergies occur to cause serious health problems. But, hopefully, what we have outlined in this book gives you a strong sense of how much evidence already exists to document the TDOS Syndrome.

AFTERWORD: NOW WHAT?

The powerful combination of forces that undermine our ability to live healthier, longer, is also stealing our ability to maximize our quality of life potential. The result of this internal storm is a steep decline in our health, including the epidemic of toxicity in our bodies from chemicals and nutritionally deficient food. We are bursting at the seams, both out of our clothes and our stress levels. Conventional dieting (counting calories) and exercise simply aren't enough, given what we now know about the assault on our bodies and health.

We hope that this book has awakened you to the stark reality we all potentially face when toxicity, nutrient deficiency, being overweight, and chronic stress combine to create the TDOS Syndrome. With awareness, you will be in a powerful position to initiate an entirely New Health Conversation, based on a clear vision of the four co-factors. No single idea, factor, process, or protocol can defeat the TDOS Syndrome. Conventional interventional protocols are simply ill-equipped to identify, much less, treat, this syndrome in any effective way.

There will always be a need for excellent medical and surgical care, along with technological advancements in diagnosis and treatment of disease. But the use of these procedural interventions is depleting resources away from preventive care. Traditional procedural interventions consume 80 percent of our precious health-care resources and treat only 20 percent of the patients who have fallen victim to a "sick" system.

Our modus operandi is to bandage the same chronic conditions over and over again. The same chronic patients return repeatedly for additional heart stents, multiple coronary bypass surgeries, and more alleged wonder drugs. The system is broken, according to both the heads of Medicare and Medicaid. There simply won't be enough money in the future to pay for this overwhelming health decline. We can only repair the body so many times before the repairs no longer work. But do not lose hope. Now is the time for stepping into a place of radical responsibility to follow an inspired regimen of preventive care-taking, for all aspects of our health.

The challenge we now face is that the TDOS Syndrome operates in stealth mode, virtually invisible, at least as far as most of the traditional health-care system is concerned. We must initiate a change in our health-care conversation in order to help us—and future generations—live healthier lives. That is one reason why we have written two separate books: one elucidating the problem, and the other detailing its solutions.

In our first book, the one you have just finished reading, we defined the TDOS Syndrome's complex and interconnected co-factors (the problem). In science, unless you can understand and identify the totality of a problem, it is impossible to discover a solution. In our second book, *The TDOS Solutions*, we will offer you revolutionary, comprehensive, and interconnected approaches to treat, prevent, and survive the TDOS Syndrome.

In our next book, we will share at length what Robert Lawrence Friedman calls "stress hardiness." Individuals who possess this seem to avoid many of the worst stress symptoms. Friedman points out specific practices that can be used, including expressing gratitude and reframing negatives into positives. We will also introduce you to David Dubin, MD, and his research with Direct Neurofeedback, an exciting new breakthrough in lowering stress in the human body. In addition, we will outline a variety of other suggestions to help minimize the effects of the four co-factors of the TDOS Syndrome.

These solutions will allow you to maximize your quality of life potential, and quite possibly extend your lifespan, as you learn to master the steps that we ourselves have already researched and tried out successfully in practice. Among the many healing tools and techniques we provide, you will learn how to:

- detoxify your body safely and effectively
- fortify yourself with quality nutrients to remedy your deficiencies
- release excess weight without relying on traditional diets and exercise programs
- relieve chronic stress using natural non-drug approaches to relaxation

We will empower you with the keys to using a holistic and synergistic solution that revolves around the concept of nutritional fasting, a remarkable program to simultaneously deliver nutrients, release toxins, and shed pounds. You will see how reducing calories in your diet, *not reducing nutrients*, energizes your health, because nutritional density is the key to weight management. You will learn in detail how and why nutritional fasting works, with a step-by-step guide to doing it on your own. We will show you how to maintain this new lifestyle momentum to achieve your health goals. And much more! We feel confident that the nutritional approach we have identified through intensive research, and trial and error, will transform your health and your life for the better.

Notes

Introduction

1. "Breast Cancer Facts & Figures 2013–14," American Cancer Society. http://www.cancer.org/acs/groups/content/@research/documents/document/acspc-042725.pdf

2. "America's Children and the Environment: Measures of Contaminants, Body Burdens, and Illnesses," Environmental Protection Agency. 2011.

3. "Reducing Environmental Cancer Risk: What We Can Do Now," President's Cancer Panel. May 2010.

4. "Deaths from Cardiovascular Disease Increase Globally," Institute for Health Metrics and Evaluation. http://www.healthdata.org.

5. Ezzat M. et al., "Trends in Adult Body-Mass Index In 200 Countries from 1975 To 2014: A Pooled Analysis of 1698 Population-Based Measurement Studies with 19.2 Million Participants." The Lancet (April 2016).

6. Global Report on Diabetes, 2016," World Health Organization, http://www.who.int/diabetes/global-report/en/

7. "2016 Alzheimer's Disease Facts and Figures," Alzheimer's Association. http://www.alz.org/facts/

8. "Parkinson's Is on the Rise," Parkinson's Disease Foundation. http://www.pdf.org.

9. Chandra A. et al., "Fertility, Family Planning, and Reproductive Health of U.S. Women," National Center for Health Statistics. Vital and Health Statistics, 2005.

10. "Vital Signs: Asthma Prevalence, Disease Characteristics and Self-Management Education—United States, 2001–2009," U.S. Centers for Disease Control and Prevention. Morbidity and Mortality Weekly Report, 2011.

11. Boyle C. et al., "Trends in the Prevalence of Developmental Disabilities in U.S. Children, 1997-2008", Pediatrics (2011).

12. "Pediatric Non-Alcoholic Fatty Liver Disease," American Liver Foundation. Shikha Sundaram, MD, http://www.liverfoundation. org.

13. Statistic Brain Research Institute, American Institute of Stress. New York, Oct. 19, 2015. http://www.statisticbrain.com/stress-statistics/

Chapter 1: Co-Factor T—Toxicity

14. "CDC Fourth National Report on Human Exposure to Environmental Chemicals," Centers for Disease Control and Prevention. www.cdc.gov/biomonitoring/pdf/FourthReport_UpdatedTablesFeb2015.pdf

15. Ibid.

16. Guergana Mileva Stephanie L. Baker, Anne T.M. Konkle, and Catherine Bielajew,"Bisphenol-A: Epigenetic Reprogramming and Effects on Reproduction and Behavior." International Journal of Environmental Research and Public Health. 2014 Jul; 11(7): 7537-7561. Published online 2014 Jul 22. doi: 10.3390/ijerph110707537

17. "Chemicals and Our Health," Safer Chemicals, Healthy Families. http://saferchemicals.org/health-report/.

18. American Lung Association, "Toxic Air: The Case for Cleaning Up Coal-Fired Plants," March 2011.

19. "Body Burden: The Pollution in People." Environmental Working Group. www.ewg.org/sites/bodyburden/findings.php.

20. http://www.ewg.org/research/body-burden-pollution-newborns

21. Goodson W.H. et al., "Assessing The Carcinogenic Potential of Low-Dose Exposures to Chemical Mixtures in the Environment: The Challenge Ahead," *Carcinogenesis* (June 2015).

22. Flora S.J., "Arsenic and Dichlorvos: Possible Interaction Between Two Environmental Contaminants," *Journal of Trace Elements in Medicine and Biology* (May 2016).

23. Chen C. et al., "The Synergistic Toxicity of the Multiple Chemical Mixture: Implications for Risk Assessment in the Terrestrial Environment." *Environment International* (April 2015).

24. Ledoigt G. et al., "Synergistic Health Effects Between Chemical Pollutants and Electromagnetic Fields." *Reviews on Environmental Health* (2015).

25. Boobis A. et al., "Critical Analysis of Literature on Low-Dose Energy for Use in Screening Chemical Mixtures for Risk Assessment." *Critical Reviews in Toxicology* (May 2011).

26. Eriksson P. et al., "Polybrominated Diphenyl Ethers, A Group of Brominated Flame Retardants, Can Interact with Polychlorinated Biphenyls in Enhancing Developmental Neurobehavioral Defects," *Toxicology Sciences* (December 2006).

27. Lau K. et al., "Synergistic Interactions Between Commonly Used Food Additives in a Developmental Neurotoxicity Test." *The Journal of Toxicological Sciences* (March 2006).

28. Lee D.H. et al., "A Strong Dose-Response Relation Between Serum Concentrations of Persistent Organic Pollutants and Diabetes. Results from the National Health and Examination Survey 1999-2002," *Diabetes Care* (2006).

29. http://www.motherjones.com/tom-philpott/2013/02/meat-industry-still-gorging -antibiotics

Chapter 2: Co-Factor D—Deficiency of Nutrition

30. "Acid Rain Study Reaches Milestone, Confirms Soil Nutrient Depletion." Soil Science Society of America. December 2003. http://www.eurekalert.org/pub_releases/2004-03/uom-ars032604.php

31. "The Rio Earth Summit: Summary of the United Nations Conference on Environment and Development." November 1992. http://publications.gc.ca/Collection-R/LoPBdP/BP/bp317-e.htm

32. Mayer A.M., "Historical Changes in the Mineral Content of Fruits and Vegetables." *British Food Journal* (1997).

33. Davis D.R. et al., "Changes in USDA Food Composition Data for 43 Garden Crops, 1950 to 1999." *Journal of American College of Nutrition* (2004).

34. "What If the World's Soil Runs Out?" World Economic Forum. Dec. 14, 2012. http://world.time.com/2012/12/14/what-if-the-worlds-soil-runs-out/

35. Welch R.M., "The Impact of Mineral Nutrients in Food Crops on Global Human Health." *Plant and Soil* (2002).

36. Udo de Haes H.A. et al., "Scarcity of Micronutrients in Soil, Feed, Food, and Mineral Reserves." Dutch Ministry of Agriculture and Foreign Trade. September 2012. http://www.iatp.org/files/scarcity of micronutrients.pdf.

37. Lathrop P.J. and Leung H.K., "Thermal Degradation and Leaching of Vitamin C from Green Peas During Processing." *Journal of Food Science* (2006).

38. Sullivan J.F. et al., "Loss of Amino Acids and Water Soluble Vitamins During Potato Processing." *Journal of Food Science* (2006).

39. Lopez-Berenguer C. et al., "Effects of Microwave Cooking Conditions on Bioactive Compounds Present in Broccoli Inflorescenes," *Journal of Agricultural Food Chemistry* (November 2007).

40. Smith-Spangler C. et al., "Are Organic Foods Safer or Healthier Than Conventional Alternatives? A Systematic Review," *Annals of Internal Medicine* (September 2012).

41. Baranski M. et al., "Higher Antioxidant and Lower Cadmium Concentrations and Lower Incidence of Pesticide Residues in Organically Grown Crops: A Systematic Literature Review and Meta-Analyses," *British Journal of Nutrition* (September 2014).

42. Smith-Spangler C. et al., "Are Organic Foods Safer or Healthier Than Conventional Alternatives? A Systematic Review," *Annals of Internal Medicine* (September 2012).

43. Baranski M. et al., "Higher Antioxidant and Lower Cadmium Concentrations and Lower Incidence of Pesticide Residues in Organically Grown Crops: A Systematic Literature Review and Meta-Analyses," *British Journal of Nutrition* (September 2014).

44. Kirstensen M. et al., "Effect of Plant Cultivation Methods on Content of Major and Trace Elements in Foodstuffs and Retention in Rats," *Journal of the Science of Food and Agriculture* (2008).

45. Bourre J.M., "Effects of Nutrients (in Food) on the Structure and Function of the Nervous System: Update on Dietary Requirements for Brain. Part 1: Micronutrients." *Journal of Nutrition Health and Aging* (Sep-Oct. 2006).

46. Bailey RL. et al., "The Epidemiology of Global Micronutrient Deficiencies." *Annals of Nutrition Metabolism* (2015).

47. Welch R.M., "The Impact of Mineral Nutrients in Food Crops on Global Human Health." *Plant and Soil* (2002).

48. Fayet-Moore F. et al., "Micronutrient Status in Female University Students: Iron, Zinc, Copper, Selenium, Vitamin B12 And Folate," *Nutrients* (November 2014).

49. Ter Borg S. et al., "Micronutrient Intakes and Potential Inadequacies of Community-Dwelling Older Adults: A Systematic Review," *British Journal of Nutrition* (April 2015).

50. Ward E., "Addressing Nutritional Gaps with Multivitamin and Mineral Supplements." *Nutrition Journal* (July 2014).

51. "http://www.seaagri.com/docs/arden_anderson.pdf"

52. http://www.news.cornell.edu/stories/2006/03/slow-insidious-soil-erosion-threatens-human-health-and-welfare.

53. Carlton J.B., "Prevalence of Micronutrient Deficiency in Popular Diet Plans." *Journal International Society of Sports Nutrition* (June 2010).

Chapter 3: Co-Factor O—Overweight

54. "It's Official: Every State in America Is Too Fat," *The Washington Post*, Sept. 24, 2015.

55. http://www.npr.org/blogs/health/2010/04/too fat to fight obesity.html.

56. Wang Y. et al., "Will All Americans Become Overweight or Obese? Estimating The Progression and Cost of the US Obesity Epidemic," *Obesity* (October 2008).

57. Zhang Y. et al., "Trends in Overweight and Obesity Among Rural Children and Adolescents from 1985 to 2014 in Shandong, China," *European Journal of Preventive Cardiology* (April 2016).

58. Ezzati M. et al., "Trends in Adult Body-Mass Index in 200 Countries From 1975 to 2014: A Pooled Analysis of 1698 Population-Based Measurement Studies with 19.2 Million Participants," *The Lancet* (April 2016).

59. http://www.nhs.uk/LiveWell/over60s/Pages/The-top-five-causes-of-premature-death.aspx

60. "Deadly Diabetes in Unrelenting March." BBC News. April 6, 2016.

61. Stel J. Legler, "The Role of Epigenetics in the Latent Effects of Early Life Exposure to Obsesogenic Endocrine Disrupting Chemicals." *Journal of Endocrinology* (October 2015).

62. Elizabeth Grossman, "Chemicals May Play Role in Rise in Obesity," *The Washington Post*, March 12, 2007.

63. Kaati G. et al., "Transgenerational Response to Nutrition, Early Life Circumstances and Longevity," *European Journal of Human Genetics* (2007).

64. Fothergill E. et al., "Persistent Metabolic Adaptation 6 Years After 'The Biggest Loser' Competition," *Obesity* (May 2016).

65. Gina Kolata, "After 'The Biggest Loser,' Their Bodies Fought to Regain Weight," *The New York Times*, May 2, 2016.

66. Gauthier MS. et al., "The Metabolically Healthy But Obese Phenotype Is Associated with Lower Plasma Levels of Persistent Organic Pollutants As Compared to the Metabolically Abnormal Obese Phenoytypes," *The Journal of Clinical Endocrinology & Metabolism* (2014).

67. Roos V. et al. "Circulating Levels of Persistent Organic Pollutants in Relation to Visceral And Subcutaneous Adipose Tissue By Abdominal MRI," *Obesity* (February 2013).

68. Lee DH. et al., "Associations of Persistent Organic Pollutants with Abdominal Obesity in the Elderly: The Prospective Investigation of the Vasculature in Uppsala Seniors Study," *Environment International* (April 2012).

69. Suarez-Lopez JR. et al. "Persistent organic pollutants in young adults and changes in glucose metabolism over a 23-year follow-up," *Environ Res.* (February 2015).

70. Tsuneyama K. et al., "Neonatal Monosodium Glutamate Treatment Causes Obesity, Diabetes, and Macrovesicular Steatohepatitis with Liver Nodules in DIAR Mice," *Journal of Gastroenterology and Hepatology* (September 2014).
71. http://www.nhlbi.nih.gov/guidelines/obesity/BMI/bmicalc.htm
72. http://www.thefiscaltimes.com/Articles/2014/06/19/Budget-Busting-US-Obesity-Costs-Climb-Past-300-Billion-Year#sthash.TWz610IK.dpu

Chapter 4: Co-Factor S—Stress

73. Cooney C.M., "Stress-Pollution Interactions: An Emerging Issue in Children's Health Research." *Environnental Health Perspectives* (October 2011).
74. http://www.apa.org/news/press/releases/stress/2012/impact.aspx?item=2
75. Talbott, Shawn M., *The Cortisol Connection: Why Stress Makes You Fat and Ruins Your Health–and What You Can Do about It* (Alameda, CA: Hunter House, 2002).
76. https://www.nlm.nih.gov/medlineplus/ency/article/004000.htm
77. http://www.oprah.com/health/Dr-Perricone-on-Stress-and-Cortisol
78. http://www.ncbi.nlm.nih.gov/pubmed/18200815
79. "Being Overweight Linked to Excess Stress Hormones After Eating," *The Endocrine Society* (June 15, 2013). http://www.eurekaalert.org/pub_releases/2013-06/tes-bol061513.php
80. Manenschijin L. et al., "High Long-Term Cortisol Levels, Measured in Scalp Ha Are Associated with a History of Cardiovascular Disease," *The Journal of Clinic Endocrinology & Metabolism* (May 2013).
81. Kvamme J.M. et al., "Risk of Malnutrition and Zinc Deficiency in Community-Living Elderly Men and Women: The Tromo Study," *Public Health Nutrition* (August 2015).
82. Olstad DL. et al., "Hair Cortisol Levels, Perceived Stress and Body Mass Index in Women and Children Living in Socioeconomically Disadvantaged Neighbo hoods: The READI Study," *Stress* (March 2016).
83. Mouchacca J. et al., "Associations Between Psychological Stress, Eating, Physic Activity, Sedentary Behaviours and Body Weight Among Women: A Longitu Study." *BCM Public Health* (September 2013).
84. Tomes SJ. et al., "Does Stress Induce Salt Intake?" *British Journal of Nutrition* (June 2010).
85. Shankardass K. et al., "Parental Stress Increases the Effect of Traffic-Related Pollution on Childhood Asthma Incidence," *Proceedings of the National Acaer of Sciences* (July 2009).
86. Cooney C.M., "Stress-Pollution Interactions: An Emerging Issue in Children Health Research," *Environmental Health Perspectives* (October 2011).

Suggested Reading

Baillie-Hamilton, Paula. Toxic Overload: *A Doctor's Plan for Combating the Illnesses Caused by Chemicals in Our Foods, Our Homes, and Our Medicine Cabinets.* New York: Avery, 2005. Print.

Batmanghelidj, F. *Water. For Health, for Healing, for Life: You're Not Sick, You're Thirsty!* New York: Grand Central Life & Style, 2012. Print.

Batmanghelidj, F. *Your Body's Many Cries for Water: You're Not Sick; You're Thirsty: Don't Treat Thirst with Medications.* Falls Church, VA: Global Health Solutions, 2008. Print.

Chevat, Richie, and Michael Pollan. *The Omnivore's Dilemma: The Secrets Behind What You Eat.* New York: Dial, 2009. Print.

Fitzgerald, Randall. *The Hundred-year Lie: How Food and Medicine Are Destroying Your Health.* New York: Dutton, 2006. Print.

Hyman, Mark, M.D. *The UltraMind Solution: Fix Your Broken Brain By Healing Your Body First.* N.p.: Scribner, 2008. Print.

Kaufman, Francine Ratner. *Diabesity: A Doctor and Her Patients on the Front Lines of the Obesity-diabetes Epidemic.* New York: Bantam, 2006. Print.

Kaufman, Francine Ratner. *Diabesity: The Obesity-diabetes Epidemic That Threatens America—and What We Must Do to Stop It.* New York: Bantam, 2005. Print.

Kessler, David A. *The End of Overeating: Taking Control of the Insatiable American Appetite.* Emmaus, PA: Rodale, 2009. Print.

Lassek, William D., and Steven J. C. Gaulin. *Why Women Need Fat: How "Healthy" Food Makes Us Gain Excess Weight and the Surprising Solution to Losing It Forever.* New York: Hudson Street, 2012. Print.

Moss, Michael. *Salt, Sugar, Fat: How the Food Giants Hooked Us.* New York: Random House, 2013. Print.

Index

A

Abdominal fat, impact, 113–114

Abdominal stress fat, impact, 115

Absorption (reduction), toxins (impact), 52

Acid rain, 56

Acute toxicity, 20

Addictive drugs, processed food chemistry (relationship), 64–67

Aging
    acceleration, 118
    infirmities, trace element deficiencies (impact), 58

Agricultural practices, impact, 47–51

Air
    breathing, toxin entry process, 21–22
    pollution, 23

Alzheimer's disease
    copper deficiency, impact, 58
    rates, increase, 1
    statistics, 4

Anabolic hormones, secretion, 117

Anderson, Arden, 62

Annals of Internal Medicine (organic food findings), 55

Anti-aging, studies, 119

Antibiotics, presence, 29–30

Antioxidants, impact, 35

Arsenic, 51, 57

Association of American Medical College (AAMC), Center for Workforce Studies, 38

Asthma
    development, 122
    statistics, 4

Attention deficit hyperactivity disorder (ADHD)
    food additives, impact, 28
    iron deficiency, impact, 58

B

Bacteria, role, 51

Balanced diet, 62

Beauty products, application (toxin entry process), 24

Behavior, Vitamin B12 deficiencies (impact), 58

Big Food industry, impact, 65

Biological toxicants, impact, 20

Biomarkers, study, 60

Birth defects, toxins (impact), 25

Bisphenol A, health impact, 17

Blood
    CDC tests, 15
    cortisol levels, presence, 115
    POP level (increase), long-term weight loss (impact), 85–86
    sugar, management, 116

Body
    abuse, limits, 30–31
    anabolic metabolism state, 117
    chemicals, presence, 19
    detoxification, 125
    mechanism, 9
        metabolism, magnesium (relationship), 58

About the Authors

Peter Greenlaw has conducted more than 1,500 lectures around the world on health topics and the ideas he presents in this book. He has been the featured speaker at the AutismOne conferences in 2014 and 2015, a frequent speaker at the CEO Club of New York City, and a guest on many television programs in such cities as Washington, DC, Los Angeles, San Francisco, Portland, and Kansas City. Greenlaw's first TV show, *The New Health Conversation*, aired on Rocky Mountain PBS, where he introduced a fresh approach to health, diet, nutrition, and TDOS. He will be the central figure in an upcoming television pilot being filmed by award-winning director Douglas Freel titled *The Greenlaw Report™*.

Nicholas Messina, MD, became a board certified family physician in 1985. He was a solo practitioner from 1985-1994. He formed a group family practice in 1994. During this time Dr. Messina was the Deputy Director of Family Practice for St. Joseph Hospital in Stamford, Connecticut, and he served on several hospital committees. In 1997 he became the Medical Director for a Complementary Wellness Center in Norwalk, Connecticut. In 1999 he became the medical director for an Independent Clinical Research Facility in Mesa, Arizona. He has been the Principal Investigator on numerous clinical trials involving many of the Fortune 500 Pharmaceutical companies. The trials included medications for arthritis, diabetes, depression, obesity, chronic pain, generalized anxiety, and other conditions. He also served as the Vice Chairman of the Board for an Independent Ethics Committee (IRB), overseeing pharmaceutical research to ensure sound scientific design and subject safety. He has been published in peer reviewed medical journals and has written articles on health related issues for several magazines He currently resides in Mesa, Arizona and does private consulting for the Healthcare, Pharmaceutical, and Financial industries.

Drew Greenlaw graduated from the University of Colorado with a degree in English. He currently lives in Colorado with his wife and three kids. Drew started working with his father, Peter, eight years ago. The two collaborated on a research project to build a case against toxins because of their effects on the human body. This early research would set the stage for the discovery of the TDOS Syndrome®. Drew continues to work behind the scenes on research and development for the new show *The Greenlaw Report™*, as well as their website www.PeterGreenlaw.com. The intention of both the show and website are to provide additional solutions as well as solution providers to further help and educate people on the current state of health and wellness.